The Maxillary Sinus

The Maxillary Sinus
and its Dental Implications

David A. McGowan, MDS (QUBelf), PhD(Lond), FDSRCS(ENG), FFDRCS(Ire), FDSRCPS(Glasg)
Professor of Oral Surgery, Glasgow Dental Hospital and School

Prudence W. Baxter, BSc (Otago), BDS (Otago), FDSRCS (Edin)
Honorary Registrar, Glasgow Dental Hospital and School

Jacqueline James, BDS (Birm), FDSRCS (Edin)
Lecturer, Department of Oral Surgery, Glasgow Dental Hospital and School

WRIGHT

Wright
An imprint of Butterworth-Heinemann Ltd
Linacre House, Jordan Hill, Oxford OX2 8DP

$\mathcal{R}$ A member of the Reed Elsevier group

OXFORD   LONDON   BOSTON
MUNICH   NEW DELHI   SINGAPORE   SYDNEY
TOKYO   TORONTO   WELLINGTON

First published 1993

British Library Cataloguing in Publication Data
A catalogue record for this book is available from
the British Library.

ISBN 0 7236 0813 X

**Library of Congress Cataloguing in Publication
Data**
A catalogue record for this book is available from
the Library of Congress.

Composition by Genesis Typesetting, Rochester, Kent
Printed in Great Britain by Martin's of Berwick-upon-Tweed

Contents

Preface

The closeness of the maxillary sinus to the upper teeth dictates that dentists must understand its anatomy and physiology and be able to distinguish the effects of sinus disease from those of dental disease. If unfortunate enough to penetrate the sinus during dental treatment, they should be able to minimize the damage caused, and it is imperative to recognize the early signs of covert neoplastic sinus disease.

The aim of this book is to provide the background knowledge required for these purposes in a convenient form. We hope it will be helpful to students and practitioners at all levels of experience, but perhaps particularly so to those studying the subject in depth for the basic science and general parts of the Dental Fellowship examinations.

We freely acknowledge our debt to the editors and authors of *Scott-Brown's Otolaryngology*, Volumes 1 and 4 (Kerr, 1987), and recommend them to those seeking an authoritative and encyclopaediac treatment of the whole range of nasal and paranasal sinus disease.

Fickling (1957) and Harrison (1961) refer to some quaint historical accounts of sinus perforation during tooth extraction which highlight the alarm aroused by this accident in both patient and surgeon. Unfortunately, similar feelings still arise today unless the problem is met with the confidence of understanding. According to Reading, Harrison and Dinsdale (1955), the dental surgeon regards the maxillary sinus as 'a dark and mysterious country which he fears to explore'. Our aim is to reduce the fear by dispelling the mystery.

References

Fickling, B. W. (1957) Oral Surgery involving the maxillary sinus. *British Dental Journal*, **103**, 199–214

Harrison, D. F. N. (1961) Oro-antral fistula. *British Journal of Clinical Practice*, **15**, 169–174

Kerr, A. G. (ed.) (1987) *Scott-Brown's Otolaryngology*, Vol. 1 (ed. D. Wright), Vol. 4 (eds I. S. Mackay and T. R. Bull), Butterworth–Heinemann, Oxford

Reading, P., Harrison, D. F. N. and Dinsdale, R. C. W. (1955) The causation, pathology and treatment of oro-antral fistula resulting from dental extraction. *Journal of Laryngology and Otology*, **69**, 729–743

Acknowledgements

Production of a book of this kind is the culmination of the efforts of many apart from the authors. Our secretaries, Mrs Isabel McGuire, Mrs Phyllis Cooke and formerly Mrs Sara Glen-Esk, have spent many hours converting scrawl to script, and we are grateful for their expertise. Our Glasgow oral surgery colleagues have been generous with their advice, experience and case material. Mrs Laetitia Brocklebank and Dr Lakshman Samaranyake helped particularly with Chapters 3 and 4, respectively. Our artist, Ms Anne Hughes, and the photographic team, led by Mr John Davies, have also been most willing and skilful. We would like particularly to acknowledge the use of the historical anatomical specimens made available to us by Dr Caroline Grigson, Osman Hill Curator, of the Odontological Museum at the Royal College of Surgeons of England. Lucy Sayer, and latterly Linda Butterworth, of our publishers have been helpful – and patient! To our families go, as always, our gratitude for their support and forbearance.

Chapter 1

Anatomy: regional, systematic and applied

The maxillary sinuses are the largest of the air-filled spaces surrounding the nose. They are paired structures located largely in the body of each maxilla, are mirror images of one another (though not always symmetrical) and are approximately pyramidal in shape (Figures 1.1 and 1.2).

The base of each pyramid is medial, its upper two-thirds being the lower half of the lateral wall of the nasal cavity, and its lower third being the palatal alveolar process; the apex is directed laterally towards the zygomatic bone and in large sinuses may extend into it. The four sloping surfaces connecting the base to the apex are: the roof of the sinus, which forms part of the orbital floor and slopes down laterally; the buccoalveolar surface or floor, which slopes up laterally; the facial surface, which faces anterolaterally; and the infratemporal surface facing posterolaterally. The sloping walls, except for the roof which receives a contribution from the lacrimal bone near its anteromedial angle, are formed entirely from the maxilla. Other bones always contribute to the base and occasionally to the apex.

Examination of a dried skull by holding a torch to the orbital floor will demonstrate the outline of the sinus and its close relationship to the anterior ethmoid air cells.

As the walls consist largely of thin bone a tumour originating within the sinus may expand up into the orbit, down into the mouth (usually the buccoalveolar process), posteriorly into the pterygopalatine fossa, or the infratemporal (pterygoid) region, forwards on to the cheek, or medially into the nasal cavity. Extraction of upper posterior teeth may damage the floor and trauma may fracture its walls.

The sinuses are usually, but not always, equal in size, and rarely one sinus may be completely absent. Their ostia open high up through the medial wall into the middle meatus of the nose (Figure 1.2). Understanding the variation of the site and orientation of the ostium is important in endoscopic sinus surgery (May, Sobol and Korzec, 1990). Bony septa may be present in the maxillary sinuses and are sometimes complete, forming smaller accessory sinuses (Miles, 1973).

The earliest recorded description of the maxillary sinus appears to be the drawings and notes of Leonardo da Vinci in 1489 (Fickling, 1957). Vesalius included a description in his *De Humani Corporis Fabrica*, published in 1543, the work which finally supplanted the teachings of Galen, the ancient Greek. Nathaniel Highmore described the sinus in his *Corporis Humani Disquisitio Anatomica* in 1651. Part of his description (quoted by Fickling, 1957) reads: 'The bone which encloses it and separates it from the sockets of the teeth does not much exceed a piece of wrapping paper in thickness.' He also describes what

Figure 1.1 (a) Coronal and (b) axial CT scans showing the shape and relations of the maxillary sinus

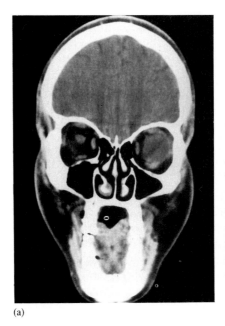
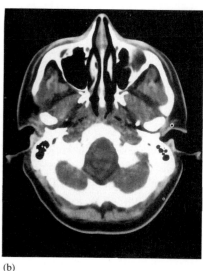

(a)   (b)

may well be the earliest recorded case of oroantral fistula. The description is quoted by Harrison (1971) as follows:

> The lower surface of this cavity (Antrum Genae) is very thin and frequently, upon drawing a tooth, is taken along with it, whereby the cavity is opened into the mouth. A gentlewoman who had had the Dens Caninus drawn on account of an inveterate defluction of sharp humours, on thrusting a silver bodkin into the alveolus, was exceedingly frightened to find it pass, as it did, almost to her eyes. Upon further trial with a small feather stript of its plume she was so terrified as to consult a doctor and others, imagining nothing less than it had gone to her brain. But they, considering the circumstances, found that the feather had doubled only in this cavity.

Cowper wrote, in his *Anatomy of Humane Bodies* in 1698:

> This cavity is called Antrum Maxillae Superioris: by some called Antrum Highmorianum for what reason I know not since 'twas described long before Dr. Highmore as appears by Vesalius, Colombus, Bauhinus etc.

Perhaps Cowper was jealous of the fame of Highmore, but despite his acerbic remarks the sinus is known by some anatomists as the 'antrum of Highmore' to this day and the term 'antrum' is current clinical usage. Highmore may not have been the first to describe the sinus, but it was perhaps because he implicated it in chronic suppuration that his name was fixed in the minds of generations of students; an early example of the power of the applied approach to anatomy! Cowper himself described a technique of drainage of sinus infection by extracting a molar tooth that was still practised up until the twentieth century (Fickling, 1957).

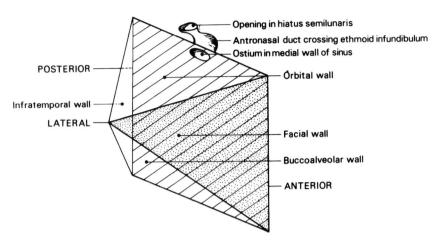

Opening in hiatus semilunaris
Antronasal duct crossing ethmoid infundibulum
Ostium in medial wall of sinus
POSTERIOR
Orbital wall
Infratemporal wall
LATERAL
Facial wall
Buccoalveolar wall
ANTERIOR

Figure 1.2 Diagram of the right maxillary sinus including the antronasal duct viewed from the anterolateral aspect

Development and age changes

During the fourth week of embryonic life the dorsal portion of the first pharyngeal arch forms the maxillary process. This extends forwards beneath the developing eye and gives rise to the maxilla, the zygomatic and part of the temporal bone.

The maxillary sinus starts to develop at about 12 weeks (80 mm crown–rump length) as an evagination from the primitive ethmoid infundibulum in the lateral wall of the middle meatus of the corresponding nasal cavity when the nasal epithelium invades the maxillary mesenchyme (Kitamura, 1989) (Figure 1.3). The infraorbital vessels and nerves are initially in an open groove on the orbital floor but its anterior part is converted into a canal by a bony lamina growing in from the lateral side (Williams *et al.*, 1989).

At birth the maxilla is filled with deciduous tooth germs which are very close to the orbital floor so the superior dental nerves and vessels have only a short distance to travel to reach the teeth (figures 1.4a). The maxillary sinus averages 7 mm in anteroposterior length and 4 mm in height and width at this stage. It expands approximately 3 mm anteroposteriorly and 2 mm vertically each year (Sperber, 1989). Because the maxillary sinus is a mere anteroposterior groove between the inferior and middle turbinates, the sinus floor is high above the level of the floor of the nose (figure 1.5). The alveolar and orbital aspects of the maxilla gradually become separated by cancellous bone which is then resorbed as the sinus enlarges. Pneumatization of the maxilla commences just below the orbital floor. Downward growth of the maxillary sinus leaves the ostium in a position unfavourable for gravitational drainage (Figure 1.5). The maxillary sinus expands not only downwards but also forwards and backwards from its initial evagination, the site of which persists as the antronasal duct (Figure 1.2). It undergoes concurrent lateral expansion and by the end of the first year extends beneath the orbit as far as the infraorbital canal (Adams and Schofield, 1963). By the 20th month it has developed further posteriorly to the position of the rudimentary first permanent molar (Ennis, 1937); however, its growth makes no contribution to the eruption of the upper teeth (Dixon, 1986).

Figure 1.3 Coronal section of a 92 mm crown–rump length human fetus showing evagination from the middle meatus which will form the maxillary sinus distally and the ethmoid infundibulum proximally. E, evagination; IM, inferior meatus; IT, inferior turbinate; MM, middle meatus; MT, middle turbinate; MxB, maxillary bone

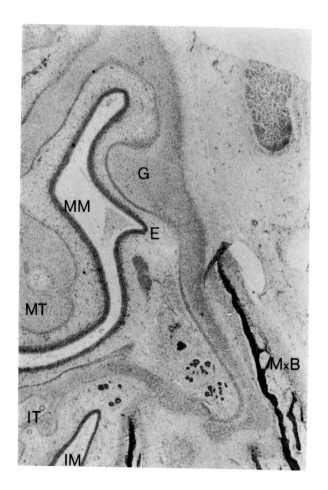

Figure 1.4 Anterior view of the facial skeleton of (a) a neonate; (b) a child aged 5; and (c) a young adult, showing the proportion of the middle third, containing the maxillary sinuses, to the rest of the face

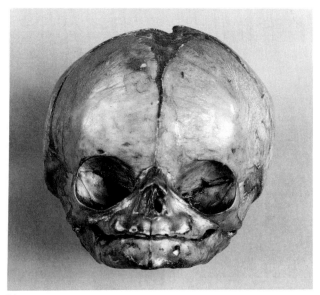

(a)

By the end of the second year the sinus has reached about half its adult size. During the third and fourth year there is a very conspicuous growth in width (Ennis, 1937), after which facial growth at the sutures is virtually complete (Sperber, 1989) (Figure 1.4b). The sinus is related to the upper deciduous second molar, the crypt of the developing upper permanent first molar, and, if it is large, to the upper deciduous first molar (Figure 1.5). As facial growth continues by surface deposition on the face, alveolar processes and palate, it is accompanied by resorption of the internal surfaces of the maxillary sinuses (Williams *et al.*, 1989). The exception is the medial wall of the sinus, where bony deposition occurs at the same rate as resorption of the lateral wall of the nose.

By the seventh year the average height is 17 mm, anteroposterior length is 27 mm and width is 18 mm (Ennis, 1937) (Figure 1.6).

The maxillary sinus grows rapidly with the facial skeleton as the permanent teeth erupt (Figures 1.4b,c and 1.7). With this increase in face height the nerves and vessels have to lengthen to continue to reach the teeth, and come to lie in canals on the facial and posterolateral walls of the sinus.

The maxillary canine usually develops in the anterolateral wall of the sinus in close proximity to the infraorbital foramen. The canine root raises a ridge on the anterior surface of the maxilla but does not indent the sinus, which lies behind it.

By the 12th year the maxillary sinus extends down to the same level as the nasal floor (Neivert, 1930) and is surgically accessible via the inferior meatus. In the adult the sinus floor is centred over the upper permanent first or second molar

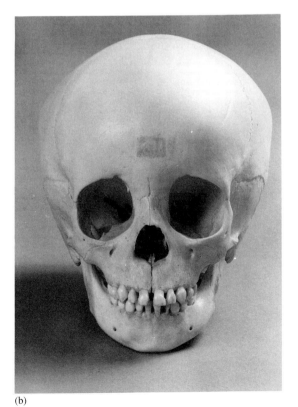

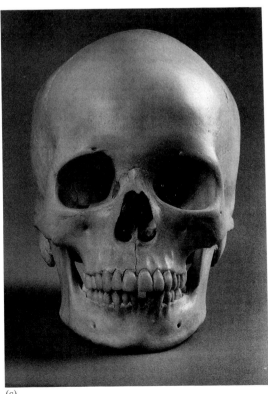

(b)   (c)

Figure 1.4 contd

Figure 1.5 Diagram showing that downward growth of the maxillary sinus leaves the ostium in a position unfavourable for gravitational drainage. From Sperber (1989)

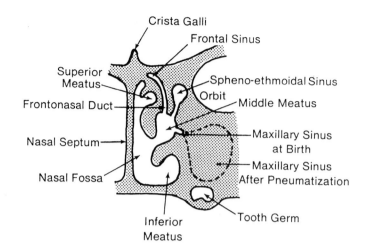

and extends to involve the premolar and possibly the canine roots, and posteriorly to involve the second and possibly the third molar roots. Facial size and shape reflect sinus dimensions (Neivert, 1930) (Figure 1.4c). The size of the adult sinus varies from person to person and even between sides in the same individual but it is approximately 35 mm in height opposite the first molar, 32 mm anteroposteriorly and 25 mm in width (Turner, 1902). Each sinus usually has a volume of about 15 ml (Neivert, 1930) but it may reach 30 ml, which equals the volume of an orbit (Swinson and McGurk, 1991).

The walls of the maxillary sinus are often uneven, the irregularities varying from shallow ridges of no practical importance to crescentic projections of considerable size that may prevent adequate surgical drainage. Occasionally a complete septum is present.

Figure 1.6 Skeleton of the left middle third of the face of a 7-year-old viewed from the lateral aspect. The facial wall of the left maxillary sinus has been removed

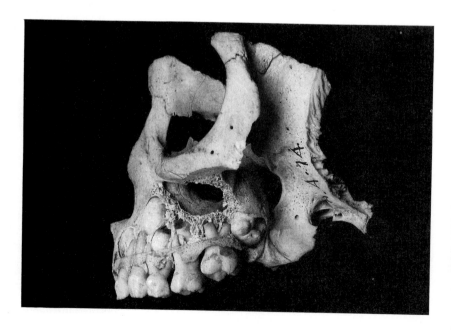

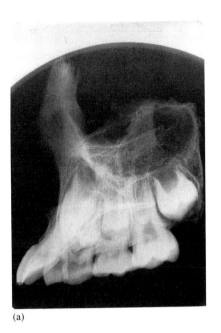

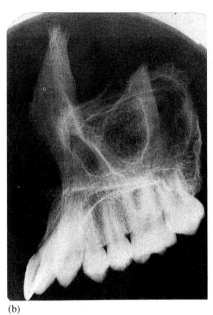

(a)   (b)

Figure 1.7 Lateral radiographs of right disarticulated maxillae in (a) an 8-year-old; and (b) a 14-year-old, showing the increase in height of the sinus with the eruption of the permanent premolars and molars

In an older edentulous maxilla, alveolar process resorption with continued sinus pneumatization may leave only a very thin layer of cortical bone separating the sinus mucosa from the oral mucosa (Figure 1.8). The middle third of the face is therefore more likely to be comminuted by trauma, and diseases of the alveolus are more likely to extend into the maxillary sinus (Dixon, 1986). Alveolar bone resorption without continued pneumatization may result in the antral floor being located level with, or even higher than the floor of the nose. While in the dentate adult the sinus floor lies more than 1 cm below the floor of the nose, in the child and in the edentulous it lies at approximately the same level (Figures 1.1a, 1.6 and 1.8).

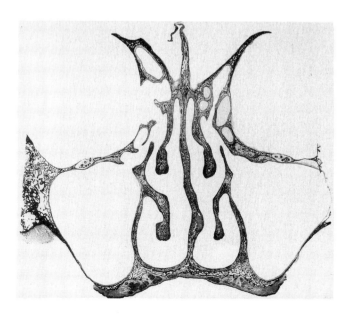

Figure 1.8 Coronal section through the mid-face showing the thin layer of bone separating the sinus mucosa from the oral mucosa in the edentulous patient. From Lund (1987)

Figure 1.9 Opened pyramid showing some internal and external relations of the maxillary sinus. AC, alveolar canal; AF, anterior fontanelle; BE, bulla ethmoidalis; BR, buccal root; CS, canalis sinuosus; DBR, distobuccal root; GPC, greater palatine canal; GPF, greater palatine foramen; IBUE, inferior surface bulla ethmoidalis; IC, inferior concha; IM, inferior meatus; IOC, infraorbital canal; IOF, infraorbital foramen; IOR, infraorbital rim; LPF, lesser palatine foramina; MBR, mesiobuccal root; MM, middle meatus; MSO, maxillary sinus ostium; NLD, nasolacrimal duct; PAP, palatal alveolar process; PF, posterior fontanelle; PPM, palatine plate of maxilla; PR, palatal root; R, root; UE, uncinate process of ethmoid; ZP, zygomatic process

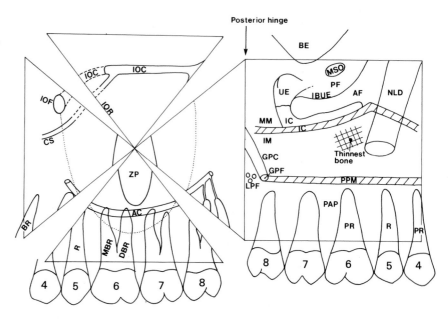

Figure 1.10 Right maxilla viewed from the posteromedial aspect with the upper bristle passing through the infraorbital groove, infraorbital canal and canalis sinuosus

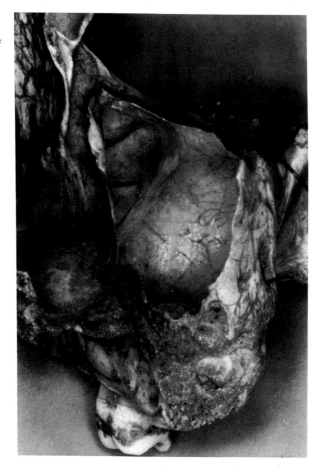

Bony walls and relations

The base and the four walls of the pyramidal sinus can be represented as a rectangle and a Maltese cross (Figure 1.9). This diagram is also reproduced in a suitable format for the construction of a three-dimensional model (Appendix 1).

Roof

This thin orbital surface extends laterally as far as the inferior orbital fissure. From examination of a disarticulated maxilla it can be seen to be formed by this bone, apart from a small contribution from the lacrimal bone near the anteromedial angle. It is smaller than the orbital floor, which also includes the orbital process of the palatine bone posteromedially, the zygomatic bone anterolaterally and the lacrimal bone medially. The orbital process of the palatine bone lies at the apex of the floor of the orbit and articulates posteriorly between the ethmoid and the maxilla.

The roof of the sinus slopes down from medial to lateral and is frequently ridged by the infraorbital groove and canal passing from the posterolateral to the facial surface and containing the infraorbital vessels and nerve. Near its midpoint this canal gives off a small branch for the anterior superior dental nerve and vessels. This sinuous branch canal descends in the orbital floor lateral to the infraorbital canal and passes into the facial wall of the maxillary sinus as the canalis sinuosus (Figure 1.10).

The most medial part of the roof forms the sloping wall of the maxilloethmoidal sinuses, from which disease may spread to the maxillary sinus.

Above the roof of the maxillary sinus is the lower part of the orbit, containing the periorbital fat, the ophthalmic artery, the zygomatic branch of the maxillary nerve, and the inferior rectus and inferior oblique muscles. The inferior oblique muscle arises near the anteromedial angle of the roof, just lateral to the opening of the nasolacrimal duct, and may make a small elevation in the sinus. The inferior rectus muscle lies above it, passing to its insertion into the sclera.

Antral infection may involve the infraorbital vessels and nerve, and malignant tumours growing in the sinus may invade the orbit and produce proptosis. Fractures of the orbital floor may result in herniation of the periorbital fat and trapping of the inferior oblique muscle. When packing an antrum, care must be taken to avoid pushing a fractured bone fragment against the ophthalmic artery, causing spasm or occlusion and subsequent blindness.

Floor

The floor of the maxillary sinus, which is curved rather than flat, is formed by the lower third of the medial wall and the buccoalveolar wall.

The buccoalveolar wall is broad medially in the depths of the alveolar process above the upper premolar and molar crowns, where it is up to 1.25 cm lower than the nasal floor. It becomes rapidly narrower laterally as it slopes up the zygomatic buttress buccal to the upper first and second molar teeth.

Roots of upper molars and premolars may ridge the floor or project into it (Figure 1.11). The floor may be subdivided by incomplete bony septa lying between the roots of the teeth, especially in the posterior part of the sinus. Neivert (1930) considered that septa were formed because the single embryological outpouching of the ethmoid infundibulum developed several finger-like projections whose distal contiguous walls did not resorb. However, Ennis (1937) thought that as blood vessels are very often within septa this may indicate that the bone containing these vessels offered more resistance to pneumatization. Root fragments displaced into the sinus during extraction may lodge in these recesses and be difficult to locate and remove. Pus contained within septal compartments may be difficult to drain (Figure 1.11).

The relationship of the maxillary teeth to the sinus varies according to the size of the sinus and the degree of pneumatization of the alveolar process, as well as with the dental age and the state of preservation of the dentition. The first and second molar roots are most commonly in close proximity to the maxillary sinus, followed by the premolar and third molar roots (Figure 1.12). Occasionally the upper canine root also encroaches upon the sinus (Ennis, 1937). Projecting roots, which make the sinus floor irregular, are usually separated from it by bone of variable thickness but sometimes by sinus mucosa alone. Periapical or periodontal infection of upper premolars and molars may therefore spread to involve the maxillary sinus (Engstrom *et al.*, 1988) and endodontic therapy or extraction of these teeth may penetrate it. Sinus infections may involve branches of the superior dental nerves to the upper molars and premolars, producing pain which is difficult to distinguish from toothache. The buccinator is attached to the alveolus overlying the upper parts of the buccal roots of the upper molars. Its muscle sheet directs pus that has perforated the mucosa and bone of the sinus floor (buccal alveolar wall) into the buccal sulcus or on to the face.

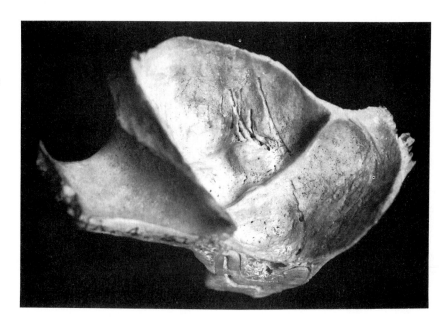

Figure 1.11 Right maxilla obliquely sectioned through an upper molar and viewed from the posterosuperior aspect, showing a septum crossing the floor of the sinus, a bony prominence over tooth roots, and the posterior superior dental neurovascular groove

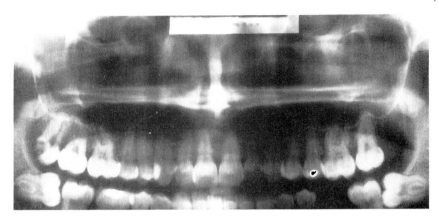

Figure 1.12 Panoramic radiograph showing the relation of the maxillary sinus to the roots of the upper premolar and molar teeth

In former times, when relief of suppurative sinus infection by drainage had a higher priority than retention of the natural teeth, Cowper's method of drainage was in vogue. This consisted of extracting the first molar and entering the sinus through the socket in order to drain pus and provide access for irrigation. First described in the early eighteenth century, this approach was still being advocated in the early twentieth century (Fickling, 1957). Fortunately it has now been abandoned in favour of access through the inferior meatus or the canine fossa, and then only in cases refractory to antibiotic therapy.

The relation between the tooth roots and the sinus floor influences orthodontic movement. Where the sinus floor is vertical and there is more bone in the direction of tooth movement there appears to be a higher degree of tipping, whereas movement through a more horizontal sinus floor is translatory (Wehrbein *et al.*, 1990).

Posterolateral wall

This wall is a curved plate which forms the anterior limit of the pterygopalatine fossa and the pterygomaxillary fissure. It also forms the oblique anterior wall of the infratemporal fossa (pterygoid region) where it is in contact with the buccal pad of fat. It is often ridged by two or three alveolar canals which pass anteriorly as they conduct the superior dental vessels and nerves from the middle of the posterolateral wall to the upper molars and the sinus mucosa.

Inferiorly is the maxillary tuberosity, which is often hollowed out by the sinus. It gives attachment to a few fibres of the medial pterygoid muscle and articulates with the pyramidal process of the palatine bone, and sometimes the lateral pterygoid plate of the sphenoid bone. Above the maxillary tuberosity posteriorly is the anterior boundary of the pterygopalatine fossa, grooved superiorly by the maxillary nerve as it passes anteriorly, veering laterally and slightly upwards above the tortuous maxillary artery. It leaves the uppermost, infratemporal part of the posterolateral wall, passing through the inferior orbital fissure and into the infraorbital groove on the orbital floor.

Facial wall

The infraorbital canal usually ridges the sinus from the thin roof to the thicker anterolateral wall as it conducts the infraorbital vessels and nerve. It ends as the funnel-shaped opening of the infraorbital foramen on the facial surface of the maxilla about 5 mm below the inferior orbital ridge. The canalis sinuosus leaves the lateral side of the orbit and passes into the facial wall of the maxillary sinus (Figure 1.10). Below the infraorbital foramen it curves medially to reach the piriform fossa (anterior bony nasal aperture) anterior to the inferior concha, and follows its lateral and then inferior margin to open near the nasal septum in front of the incisive canal. The canal contains the anterior superior dental nerve and vessels.

The canine fossa lies distal to the canine eminence and anterior to the zygomatic process of the maxilla, between the infraorbital foramen above and the alveolar process below. It is the usual site of entry into the antrum in a Caldwell–Luc operation. As the superior dental plexus of nerves traverses the canine fossa in the canalis sinuosus it may be damaged, with resultant changes in sensation of the upper anterior teeth, the adjacent periodontal ligament and the labial gingiva.

The levator labii superioris, levator labii superioris alaeque nasi and lower orbital fibres of the orbicularis oculi muscles are attached to the facial surface of the maxilla above the infraorbital foramen. Levator anguli oris is attached at the upper first premolar apex and the transverse part of nasalis at the canine apex. The muscles originating from these attachments will direct the spread of infection that penetrates the facial wall of the sinus.

Medial wall

The medial wall or base of the sinus occupies a parasagittal plane but is only partly formed by the lateral wall of the nose (Figure 1.13a,b). For descriptive purposes, it may be divided into thirds vertically. The inferior third of the medial wall is the palatal alveolar process of the maxilla (Figure 1.13c,d). The upper two-thirds of the medial wall, which also forms the lower half of the lateral wall of the nose, may be divided into two parts in relation to the inferior concha (Figures 1.13a). The part below the inferior concha is bony and forms the lateral wall of the inferior meatus. The medial wall of the sinus is indented here by the lateral bulge of the adjacent inferior meatus. The superior central portion of the inferior meatus, where the bone is thinnest, is the usual site for intranasal antrostomy. The part above the inferior concha is bony anteriorly and posteriorly but its middle part is largely composed of mucous membrane divided obliquely by the uncinate process of the ethmoid bone (Figure 1.13c).

The skeleton of the medial wall of the maxilla is complex. The bony hiatus in the posterior part of the upper two-thirds of the medial wall has its upper limit at the floor of the orbit (Figure 1.13b). It is reduced in size by contributions from the maxillary process of the inferior concha below, the perpendicular plate of the palatine bone behind, the lower border of the ethmoid labyrinth and the lateral wall of the bulla ethmoidalis above, and the inferomedial descending process of the lacrimal bone as it forms part of the nasolacrimal duct anterosuperiorly (Figure 1.13d).

The uncinate process of the ethmoid (Latin *uncinus*, a hook) is formed as a posteroinferior projection from the inferomedial wall of the anterior ethmoid air cells, starting 3 mm medial to the junction of the maxilla, lacrimal and ethmoid bones in the medial wall of the orbit. It is a laterally curving hook or J-shaped projection, the long arm of which passes obliquely from anterosuperomedial to posteroinferolateral in the lateral wall of the middle meatus to articulate with the inferior concha (Figure 1.13c). It is the junction of the long and short arms of the J which articulates with the inferior concha. The inferolateral edge of the uncinate process divides the upper anterior part of the maxillary hiatus into anteroinferior and posterosuperior parts. The medial wall of the sinus is covered with respiratory mucosa which covers the bone and comes together with the nasal mucosa to form two fontanelles, one anterior and one posterior, to occlude the maxillary hiatus. The short arm of the uncinate process projects into the medial wall of the sinus and may cause a ridge within the posterior fontanelle. The posterosuperior fontanelle itself contains an opening, the maxillary sinus ostium, which is the entrance from the antrum into the antronasal duct between the sinus and the nose (Grant, 1983)(Figure 1.14).

The maxillary sinus ostium, which is high on the medial wall of the antrum, is situated half-way between its anterior and posterior boundaries (May, Sobol and Korzec, 1990) (Figure 1.2). May and colleagues (1990) found by antroscopy that 10% of 100 patients had an accessory ostium in the posterior fontanelle, usually bilaterally. Previous reports suggested a frequency of 43% (Schaeffer, 1920), 25% (Neivert, 1930), 31% (Myerson, 1932) or 23% (Van Alyea, 1936). Accessory ostia are usually found below and behind the main ostium, sometimes in front of, but usually behind the uncinate process (Figure 1.15) (Williams *et al.*, 1989).

The ridge created by the nasolacrimal duct courses in the anterior bony part of the medial wall in front of the maxillary hiatus. The duct passes from the anterosuperomedial corner of the maxillary sinus down and slightly backwards, to open into the nose at a level approximately half-way down the medial wall of the maxillary sinus (Figures 1.10 and 1.13b,d). It may be obstructed by tumours of the sinus leading to epiphora (tears rolling down the cheek). The nasal opening of the duct is in the inferior meatus, at the junction of its anterior and middle thirds, and under cover of the inferior turbinate. Just behind it is the area of thin bone which is usually penetrated to create an antrostomy from the inferior meatus.

Posteroinferiorly there may be a convexity over the greater palatine canal as it passes down between the junction of the medial and infratemporal walls of the maxillary sinus anterolaterally and the pyramidal process (tubercule) and perpendicular plate of the palatine bone posteromedially. The greater palatine canal conveys the greater and lesser palatine vessels and nerves downwards and forwards from the pterygopalatine fossa to the single greater, and the two or three lesser, palatine foramina, respectively.

Antronasal duct

The hemispherical ethmoid bulla is formed by 1–4 middle ethmoid air cells which are, by definition, those opening on to the bulla. The hiatus semilunaris is a flat, crescent-shaped defect in the parasagittal plane within the nasal cavity. It

Figure 1.13 (a) Diagram of the medial wall of the left maxillary sinus viewed from within the sinus. U, uncinate process; E, ethmoid bone; AIF, antero-inferior fontanelle; SA, short arm of the uncinate process; PSF, postero-superior fontanelle; P, palatine bone; IC, inferior concha (b) Medial surface of a disarticulated left maxilla showing the maxillary hiatus in a 14-year-old (Figure 1.7b is a radiograph of this specimen). (c) Diagram of a coronal section passing halfway between the anterior and posterior boundaries and showing the vertical division of the sinus thirds (at line x on (a)). BE, bulla ethmoidalis; MC, middle concha; U, uncinate process; PSF, postero-superior fontanelle; AIF, anterio-inferior fontanelle; 7M, 2nd molar (d) Similar section of a skull

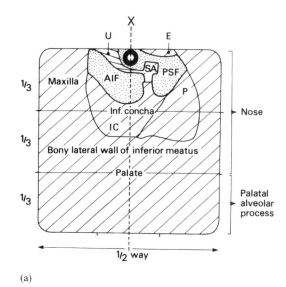

(a)

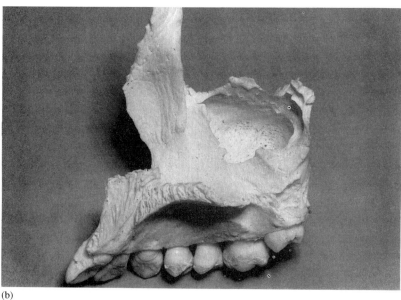

(b)

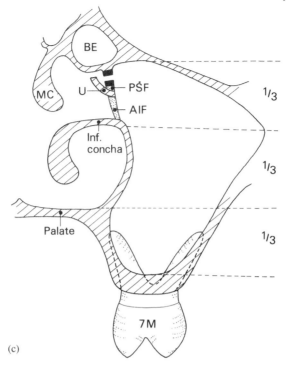

(c)

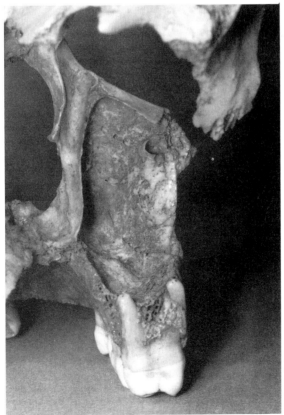

(d)

is bounded anteroinferiorly by the superior (medial) edge of the uncinate process of the ethmoid, and posterosuperiorly by the convex lower surface of the ethmoid bulla (Figure 1.14).

The ethmoid infundibulum is a funnel-shaped passage with its highest and widest part at the anterior end of the ethmoid labyrinth beneath the frontal sinus. It leads from the anterior ethmoid air cells or frontal sinus through the ethmoid labyrinth to the middle meatus. As it descends it forms a sulcus within the nasal cavity lateral to the hiatus semilunaris and medial to the medial wall of the antrum. It lies between the convex lower surface of the bulla ethmoidalis above and behind and the superolateral surface of the uncinate process of the ethmoid in front and below (Figure 1.14).

The frontal sinuses may be regarded as very large anterior ethmoid air cells which open into the middle meatus via the frontonasal duct (Figure 1.16). Kasper (1936) found, in 62% of cases, the frontonasal duct opened into the anterior part of the middle meatus (frontal recess) in front of or above the ethmoid infundibulum. The remaining 38% drained directly or indirectly via an anterior ethmoid air cell into the ethmoid infundibulum itself. Thus the ethmoid infundibulum often drains the frontal sinus as well as the anterior ethmoid air cells and the maxillary sinus. The ethmoid infundibulum is posterosuperomedial to the nasolacrimal duct, just as the middle turbinate is posterosuperomedial to the inferior turbinate (Figure 1.14).

The maxillary sinus ostium is located in the anterosuperior angle of the posterosuperior fontanelle. It lies lateral to, but at a level above the uncinate process and below the bulla of the ethmoid. It is directly below the orbit (Figure 1.13). The ostium is elliptical or hourglass-shaped, with its long axis running horizontal or anterosuperior to posteroinferior (May, Sobol and Korzec, 1990).

In 11% of cases, when the posteroinferior end of the ethmoid infundibulum is anterior to the maxillary ostial opening the sinus opens directly into the hiatus

Figure 1.14 Left parasagittal aspect of a skull viewed from the medial side, showing the complexity of the bony structure of the middle meatus. PEAC, posterior ethmoid air cell; MT, middle-turbinate; PPE, perpendicular plate of the ethmoid bone; SPF, spheno-palatine foramen; PPP, perpendicular plate of the palatine; BE, bulla ethmoidalis; MS, maxillary sinus; U, uncinate process; L, lacrimal bone; IT, inferior turbinate; MPIT, maxillary process of the inferior turbinate; CC, conchal crest of the maxilla; FPM, frontal process of the maxilla

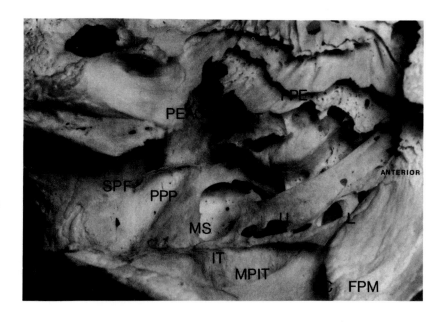

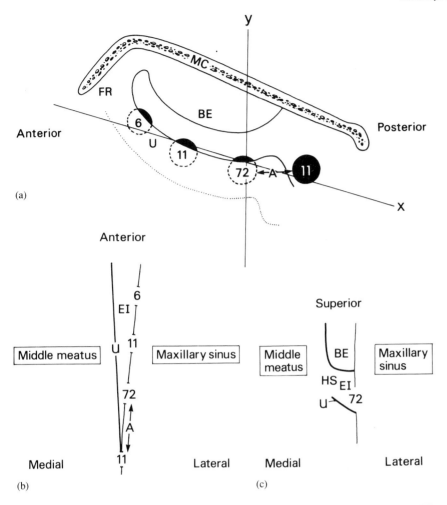

(a)

(b)

(c)

Figure 1.15 (a) Upper part of the middle meatus of the nose looking through the hiatus semilunaris into the ethmoid infundibulum, showing the positions of the maxillary sinus ostium. MC, middle concha; FR, frontal recess; BE, bulla ethmoidalis; U, uncinate process; the dimension A represents the limits of the anterior 1/3 of the ethmoidal infundibulum. (After Hollinshead, W. H. (1982). Numbers indicate percentages according to Van Aylea (1936). Scott Brown's Otolaryngology Vol. 4 Basic Sciences, Chapter 5 Anatomy of the nose and paranasal sinuses. Rhys-Evans, Fig.5.30). (b) Oblique transverse (axial) section through x to show how the ethmoid infundibulum narrows posteriorly. EI, ethmoid infundibulum; U, uncinate process; the dimension A represents the limits of the anterior 1/3 of the ethmoidal infundibulum. (c) Coronal section through y. BE, bulla ethmoidalis; HS, hiatus semilunaris; EI, ethmoid infundibulum; U, uncinate process

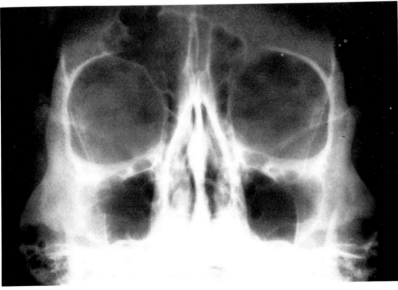

Figure 1.16 Occipitomental radiograph showing the contiguous relationship of the frontal, ethmoidal and maxillary sinuses

semilunaris. In 72% of cases, the antronasal duct opens into the posterior part of the hiatus semilunaris in the lateral wall of the middle meatus, after passing through the posterior (inferolateral) part of the ethmoid infundibulum (Figure 1.15). The antronasal duct is usually 5 mm long and curves posteriorly as it travels superomedially to the hiatus semilunaris. Its shape varies greatly (Myerson, 1932). Its nasal opening is usually oval, measuring 6 mm $\times$ 3.5 mm, at the posterior end of the hiatus semilunaris (Grant, 1983), but the anatomy of the middle meatus is also extremely variable, and so the ostium is constant in neither size nor position (Neivert, 1930). The middle turbinate, which joins the rest of the ethmoid bone at a level half-way up the orbit (i.e. at the level of the pupil), overlies the lateral wall of the middle meatus completely and makes its examination by direct vision difficult or even impossible.

Vascular supply

Arterial blood supply

The blood supply to the mucous membrane of the maxillary sinuses is rich but the sinus mucosa is not as vascular as the oral or nasal mucosa. The posterior, middle and anterior superior dental, greater palatine and sphenopalatine branches of the third part of the maxillary artery all contribute to the blood supply of the antral mucosa (Figure 1.17, Appendix 2). *Gray's Anatomy* (Williams *et al.*, 1989) states that the blood supply is from the facial as well as the infraorbital and greater palatine vessels. However, according to Neivert (1930) and Hollinshead (1982) its largest artery is a branch of the superior artery on the inferior concha which enters via the ostium. This originates from the posterior inferior lateral nasal branch of the sphenopalatine artery. Another branch of this artery enters the inferior meatus posterosuperiorly, passing inferiorly on its lateral wall to the level of the palate. It limits the posterior extent of inferior meatal antrostomy.

The maxillary artery, which is the larger terminal branch of the external carotid artery, arises in the parotid gland. Its third (pterygopalatine) part turns medially between the two heads of the lateral pterygoid and passes through the pterygomaxillary fissure into the superior part of the pterygopalatine fossa (Figure 1.17, Appendix 2). Passing laterally to medially just below the maxillary nerve, it branches into the posterior superior dental, infraorbital, greater palatine and pharyngeal arteries, the artery of the pterygoid canal and the sphenopalatine artery. All these arteries accompany branches of the maxillary nerve which also arise in the pterygopalatine fossa (Figure 1.18, Appendix 3).

The posterior superior dental artery originates from the maxillary artery as it enters the pterygopalatine fossa. It descends outside the infratemporal wall of the maxillary sinus and divides into a number of smaller branches. Some of these enter one or more bony alveolar canals on the posterior surface of the maxilla; above the apices of the upper molars they form a plexus from which branches supply the mucous membrane of the antral mucosa. These are also the arteries which maintain the vitality of the upper premolar and molar teeth.

The infraorbital artery passes anteriorly via the inferior orbital fissure to lie in the infraorbital groove in the floor of the orbit, then through the infraorbital canal to emerge from the infraorbital foramen on to the face under cover of the levator

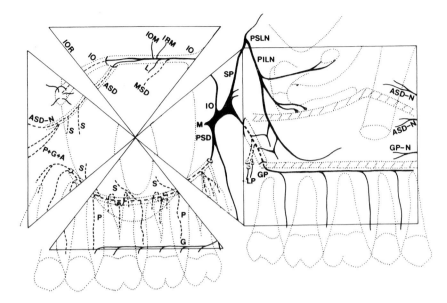

Figure 1.17 Opened pyramid showing arteries related to the maxillary sinus. A, apical arteries to teeth; ASD, anterior superior dental artery; G, arteries supplying the gingiva; GP, greater palatine artery; IO, infraorbital artery; IOM, artery to inferior oblique muscle; IOR, inferior orbital rim; IRM, artery to inferior rectus muscle; L, artery to lacrimal gland; LP, lesser palatine arteries; M, maxillary artery; MSD, middle superior dental artery; N, nasal branches; P, arteries to periodontal ligament and alveolus; PILN, posterior inferior lateral nasal branch of sphenopalatine artery; PSD, posterior superior dental artery; PSLN, posterior superior lateral nasal branches of sphenopalatine artery; S, arteries supplying antral mucosa; SP, sphenopalatine artery which enters the superior meatus;

labii superioris. Near the midpoint of its course on the roof of the maxillary sinus the infraorbital artery sends orbital branches to the inferior rectus, the inferior oblique and to the lacrimal sac. It may rarely give off a middle superior dental artery before the anterior superior dental artery. These superior dental arteries lie in neurovascular canals in the bone forming the facial wall of the sinus, in close relation to the antral mucosa which they supply before going on to supply the upper incisor and canine teeth (Williams *et al.*, 1989).

The greater palatine artery passes vertically down with the greater palatine nerve, through the greater palatine canal on the lateral side of the thin perpendicular plate of the palatine bone. In the greater palatine canal a number of branches of the greater palatine artery penetrate the perpendicular plate of the palatine bone and anastomose on the lateral nasal wall with the lateral nasal branches of the sphenopalatine artery. These help supply the posteroinferior part of the nasal cavity. Lateral branches from the greater palatine artery may supply the posteromedial area of the sinus mucosa. Anteriorly, terminal branches travel up the incisive canal to help supply the anteroinferolateral wall of the nose, but do not reach the sinus. The greater palatine artery may be damaged during bone removal in the lower posterior angle of the inferior meatus during antrostomy (Neivert, 1930).

The sphenopalatine artery leaves the pterygopalatine fossa medially through the sphenopalatine foramen to enter the superior meatus of the nose. Posterior lateral nasal branches of the sphenopalatine artery run forward on the lateral wall of the nose, particularly over the middle and inferior turbinates, to supply the mucous membrane covering the greater part of the lateral nasal wall and the medial wall of the maxillary sinus.

There are many arterial anastomoses in the region of the maxillary sinus. Just after passing through the sphenopalatine foramen, the sphenopalatine artery sends a branch across the roof of the nasal cavity which ramifies over the nasal septum. One nasopalatine or posterior septal branch passes down and forwards on the vomer to the incisive foramen, near which it anastomoses with the greater palatine artery and the septal branch of the superior labial branch of the facial artery. The infraorbital branch of the maxillary artery anastomoses with the terminal branches of the facial artery near the medial canthus, the external nasal branch of the ophthalmic artery (a branch of the internal carotid artery) on the nose, and the transverse facial branch of the superficial temporal and buccal branch of the second part of the maxillary artery above the angle of the mouth. Branches of the posterior superior dental artery and the buccal artery anastomose in the cheek, and the anterior superior dental artery connects with branches of the sphenopalatine artery.

It is this rich network of anastomotic connections which accounts for the good survival of fractured bone fragments in this part of the jaws, permits deliberate down-fracture of the maxilla without loss of the blood supply, and promotes rapid wound healing.

Venous drainage

The basic pattern of venous drainage is to the pterygoid venous plexus posteriorly, with some to the facial vein anteriorly. The distribution of veins is much more variable than that of the arteries. Veins run with the anterior, (middle) and posterior superior dental arteries in their neurovascular canals on the facial and infratemporal walls of the maxillary sinus, and also pass within the membranous fontanelles to the nasal cavity.

The anterior (and middle) superior dental veins drain superiorly into the infraorbital veins, and then posteriorly through the infraorbital canal, infraorbital groove and inferior orbital fissure to the upper part of the pterygopalatine fossa.

Tributaries of the sphenopalatine veins pass from the medial wall of the maxillary sinus via the fontanelles to the lateral wall of the nose, and leave the nasal cavity posterosuperolaterally through the sphenopalatine foramen to enter the pterygopalatine fossa.

The posterior superior dental veins drain posteriorly in the same alveolar canals as the arteries and nerves, travelling almost horizontally to exit through foramina on the posterior surface of the maxilla into the pterygopalatine fossa.

From the pterygopalatine fossa the veins draining the maxillary sinus pass laterally into the infratemporal region to enter the dense pterygoid venous plexus, which is closely related to the lateral and medial pterygoid muscles. The (anterior) facial vein sends the buccal (deep facial) vein posteriorly on the buccinator deep to the masseter and the mandibular ramus to join the plexus. This connection is important in the spread of infection.

The pterygoid plexus forms the short wide maxillary vein which enters the parotid gland and joins with the superficial temporal vein to form the retromandibular (posterior facial) vein. The retromandibular vein, which exists only within the parotid, splits into an anterior and a posterior branch. The anterior branch joins the (anterior) facial vein to form the common facial vein, which crosses the external and then the internal carotid arteries to enter the internal jugular vein in the carotid triangle.

The posterior branch of the retromandibular vein joins the posterior auricular vein on the surface of the sternocleidomastoid to form the external jugular vein.

Infection from the maxillary sinus may spread to involve the cavernous sinus via any of its draining veins. The pterygoid plexus communicates with the cavernous sinus by emissary veins passing through the foramen lacerum and foramen ovale. The infraorbital vein communicates with the facial vein through the infraorbital foramen. As the facial vein has no valves, facial muscle contraction may cause retrograde flow up towards the medial canthus of the eye through the angular vein and into its supraorbital and supratrochlear tributaries. These formative tributaries communicate with the superior and inferior ophthalmic veins, which pass between the two heads of the lateral rectus muscle and through the superior orbital fissure to the cavernous sinus. This route may be important in the spread of infection from the maxillary sinus, but the source is more likely to be the upper canine apex or the nose.

Inflammation and allergy of the nasal cavity causing venous and lymphatic congestion of the ostium results in impaired mucous drainage and secondary sinus pathology.

Lymphatic drainage

Lymphatic drainage patterns are important because infections and malignant tumours may spread along the lymphatic system.

Submucosal lymphatics of the maxillary sinus anastomose with each other, converge towards the ostium and pass through the fontanelles to unite with lymphatics of the mucous membrane of the lateral wall of the middle meatus. The well-developed lymph drainage of the lateral nasal wall is posteriorly towards the pharyngeal opening of the auditory (Eustachian) tube where the vessels form a small lymphatic plexus (Rouviere, 1938). Lymphatic vessels pierce or pass above the superior constrictor muscle to join the upper deep cervical lymph nodes, either directly or via the retropharyngeal nodes (Williams *et al.*, 1989). The retropharyngeal nodes consist of a median and two lateral groups, all lying in the buccopharyngeal fascia (Neivert, 1930) and between the pharyngeal and the prevertebral fasciae.

Lymph from the maxillary sinus does *not* drain anteriorly to join that from the face and anterior nasal cavity in draining via the submandibular lymph nodes to the upper and lower deep cervical nodes (Dixon and Hoerr, 1944). In experiments in rabbits, lymphatic drainage of the maxillary sinus was found to be slow, with all colloid material being trapped in the cervical lymph nodes and never reaching the bloodstream (Dixon and Hoerr, 1944).

The upper deep cervical lymph nodes lie along the carotid sheath in close proximity to the internal jugular vein. Most are deep to the sternomastoid muscle but a few project from its anterior border. Efferent lymphatics from the upper deep cervical lymph nodes pass to the lower deep cervical group and also directly to the jugular lymphatic trunk. The left jugular lymphatic trunk drains into the thoracic duct and the right jugular lymphatic trunk into the right lymphatic duct, from which lymph ultimately enters the venous system.

Nerve supply

General sensory innervation is from branches of the maxillary nerve, sympathetic from the superior cervical ganglion, and parasympathetic from the sphenopalatine ganglion. These fibres are distributed via the posterior and middle superior dental and infraorbital branches of the maxillary nerve (Williams *et al.*, 1989) and via the greater palatine and nasal branches from the pterygopalatine ganglion.

The respiratory mucosa of the maxillary sinus receives a dense network of adrenergic and cholinergic nerve fibres (Stammberger and Wolf, 1988), which are branches of the nerves which also supply the dental pulps of the upper teeth (Kitamura, 1989).

Sensory nerves (Figure 1.18)

The anterior superior dental nerve is everywhere closely related to the artery of the same name. It arises from the lateral side of the infraorbital nerve, near the midpoint of the infraorbital canal, 15 mm behind the infraorbital foramen (Harrison, 1971). It runs in the canalis sinuosus, forwards and downwards in the roof of the sinus lateral to the infraorbital canal. The canalis passes inferiorly then curves medially beneath the infraorbital foramen. The anterior superior dental nerve plexus supplies the roof, the facial wall and the anterior part of the medial wall of the maxillary sinus before giving off its nasal branch. This nasal branch passes through a minute canal in the lateral wall of the inferior meatus anterior to the inferior concha. It supplies an area of mucous membrane over the lower anterior region of the lateral nasal wall as high as the opening of the antronasal duct in the hiatus semilunaris. It terminates in a tiny septal branch. The anterior superior dental nerve plexus terminates by supplying the upper incisor and canine teeth and the labial gingivae.

Figure 1.18 Opened pyramid showing nerves associated with the maxillary sinus. APG, apical, periodontal ligament and gingival branches; ASD, anterior superior dental nerve; ASD-N, nasal branch of anterior superior dental nerve; GP, greater palatine nerve; IO, infraorbital nerve; LP, lesser palatine nerve; LPIN, lateral posterior inferior nasal nerve; LPSN, lateral posterior superior nasal nerve; MSD, middle superior dental nerve; MX, maxillary nerve; N, nasal branch of sphenopalatine ganglion; Na, nasal branch of the infraorbital nerve; NPC, nerve of the pterygoid canal; Pal, palpebral branches; PSD, posterior superior dental nerve; S, nerves to maxillary sinus mucosa; SL, superior labial nerves

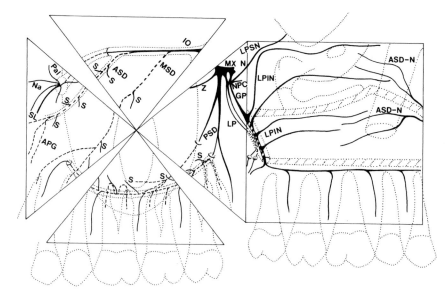

The posterior superior dental nerve arises from the maxillary nerve in the pterygopalatine fossa immediately before it enters the inferior orbital fissure. It usually divides into two, descends and pierces the posterolateral wall of the maxilla with the posterior superior dental vessels in the alveolar canals, which may project as ridges into the sinus (Williams *et al.*, 1989). It continues to descend between the mucous membrane and the bony walls of the maxillary sinus, supplying the posterolateral and inferior walls and then contributing to the molar part of the superior dental plexus.

The prevalence of the middle superior dental nerve is controversial but Harrison (1971) identified it, in 18 of 20 cadaveric maxillae, as leaving the infraorbital nerve in the infraorbital groove and running in the posterolateral or facial walls of the sinus. It supplies the antral mucosa superiorly and laterally, and contributes to the part of the superior dental plexus supplying the upper premolar teeth.

The greater palatine branch of the sphenopalatine ganglion descends in the greater palatine canal at the junction of the medial and posterolateral walls of the sinus, before emerging through the greater palatine foramen. While in the greater palatine canal it gives off posterior inferior nasal branches, which enter the nose through foramina in the perpendicular plate of the palatine bone. In addition to their general sensory function, they also supply the seromucous glands of the inferior nasal concha and the walls of the inferior and middle meatus.

The lesser palatine branches of the ganglion also pass through the greater palatine canal but emerge through the lesser palatine foramina to supply the soft palate, uvula and tonsil. Nasal branches of the pterygopalatine ganglion pass through the sphenopalatine foramen. The lower lateral posterior superior nasal nerves innervate the mucosa of the posterior part of the middle nasal concha.

All these nerves pass close to or through the sphenopalatine ganglion, so a local anaesthetic block of the ganglion will anaesthetize the maxillary sinus.

Pain arising from the maxillary sinus may be felt in the maxillary region but is sometimes perceived as involving one or more of the upper teeth. This pain is referred because the same superior dental nerves supplying the sinus mucosa supply the upper teeth.

Sympathetic

The hypothalamus controls the sympathetic nerve supply to the maxillary sinus via synapses in the intermediolateral column of the upper thoracic spinal cord and the superior cervical ganglion (Figure 1.19).

Parasympathetic

The hypothalamus regulates the parasympathetic input to the maxillary sinus via synapses in the superior salivatory nucleus and pterygopalatine (sphenopalatine) ganglion (Figure 1.20).

Anticholinergic effects of antihistamines block the parasympathetic nerves, producing a relative increase in sympathetic tone and therefore vasoconstriction and an improved airway. Destruction of the sphenopalatine ganglion, a common operation in the past for hay fever and allergic conditions, is followed by a catastrophic atrophy of the glandular tissue of the sinuses, palate and nose.

Figure 1.19 Sympathetic nerve supply to the maxillary sinus. III, third ventricle; AS, aqueduct of Sylvius; ASD, anterior superior dental nerve; CSN, cervical sympathetic nerve; DP, deep petrosal nerve; ECA, external carotid artery; GP, greater palatine nerve; H, region of hypothalamus; ICA, internal carotid artery; ICP, internal carotid plexus; IO, infraorbital nerve; MA, maxillary artery; MN, maxillary nerve; MSD, middle superior dental nerve; N, lateral posterior superior nasal branch of pterygopalatine ganglion; OC, optic chiasma; PC, pterygoid canal; PG, paravertebral ganglion of sympathetic chain; PSD, posterior superior dental nerve; SCG, superior cervical ganglion (C2–3 level); SPG, sphenopalatine ganglion; ST, sympathetic trunk; TG, trigeminal ganglion; T₁, spinal cord at level of first thoracic vertebra

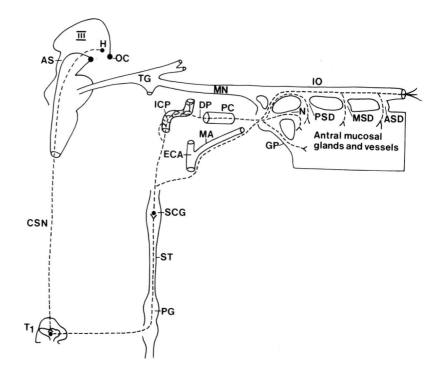

Figure 1.20 Parasympathetic nerve supply to the maxillary sinus. FC, facial canal; FL, foramen lacerum; GG, geniculate ganglion; GSPN, greater superficial petrosal nerve; IAM, internal auditory meatus; ION, infraorbital nerve; nasal branch of pterygopalatine ganglion; NI, nervus intermedius; PTB, petrous temporal bone; SSN, superior salivatory nucleus; and see Figure 1.19

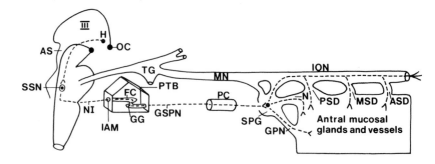

References

Adams, W. E. and Schofield, G. C. (1963) *Manual of Human Anatomy*, Vol. 1, Peryer, Christchurch, New Zealand

Cowper, C. (1698) *The Anatomy of Humane Bodies*, S. Smith and B. Walford, London, Table 92. Cited by Fickling, B. W. (1957)

Dixon, A. D. (1986) *Anatomy for Students of Dentistry*, 5th edn, Churchill Livingstone, Edinburgh

Dixon, F. W. and Hoerr, N. L. (1944) The lymphatic drainage of the paranasal sinuses. *Laryngoscope*, **54,** 165–175

Engstrom, H., Chamberlain, D., Kiger, R. and Egelberg, J. (1988) Radiographic evaluation of the effect of initial periodontal therapy on thickness of the maxillary sinus mucosa. *Journal of Periodontology* **59,** 604–698

Ennis, L. M. (1937) Roentgenographic variations of maxillary sinus and nutrient canals of maxilla and mandible. *International Journal of Orthodontia*, **23,** 173–193

Fickling, B. W. (1957) Oral surgery involving the maxillary sinus. *British Dental Journal*, **103,** 199–214

Grant, J. C. B. (1983) *Grant's Atlas of Anatomy*, 8th edn, Williams and Wilkins, Baltimore

Harrison, D. F. N. (1971) Surgical anatomy of maxillary and ethmoidal sinuses – a reappraisal. *Laryngoscope*, **81,** 1658–1664

Highmore, N. (1651) *Corporis Humani Disquisitio Anatomica*, S. Brown, The Hague, p. 226. Cited by Fickling, B. W. (1957)

Hollinshead, W. H. (1982) *Anatomy for Surgeons*, Vol. 1, 3rd edn, Harper and Row, Philadelphia, p. 261

Kasper, K. A. (1936) Nasofrontal connections: a study based on 100 consecutive dissections. *Archives of Otolaryngology*, **23,** 322–343

Kitamura, H. (1989) *Embryology of the Mouth and Related Structures*, Maruzen, Tokyo, p. 197

Lund, V. J. (1987) Surgical management of sinusitis. In *Scott-Brown's Otolaryngology*, Vol. 4, 5th edn (eds I. S. Mackay and T. R. Bull), Butterworth–Heinemann, Oxford, chap. 11

May, M., Sobol, S. M. and Korzec, K. (1990) The location of the maxillary os and its importance to the endoscopic sinus surgeon. *Laryngoscope*, **100,** 1037–1042

Miles, A. E. W. (1973) The maxillary antrum. *British Dental Journal*, **134,** 61–63

Myerson, M. (1932) The natural orifice of the maxillary Sinus. I: Anatomic studies. *Archives of Otolaryngology*, **15,** 80–91

Neivert, H. (1930) Surgical anatomy of the maxillary sinus. *Laryngoscope*, **40,** 1–4

Rouviere, H. (1938) *Anatomy of the Human Lymphatic System*, Ann Arbor, Edwards, Michigan

Schaeffer, J. P. (1920) *The Nose, Paranasal Sinuses, Nasolacrimal Passageways and Olfactory Organ in Man. A Genetic, Developmental and Anatomico-pathological Consideration*, Blakiston, Philadelphia

Sperber, G. H. (1989) *Craniofacial Embryology*, 4th edn, Wright, London, pp. 144–146

Stammberger, H. and Wolf, G. (1988) Headaches and sinus disease: endoscopic approach. *Annals of Otology, Rhinology, and Laryngology*, **97,** (Suppl. 134), 3–23

Swinson, B. D. and McGurk, M. (1991) CT estimation of orbital volume. *Journal of Dental Research*, **70,** 719

Turner, A. L. (1902) Some points in the anatomy of the antrum of Highmore. *Dental Record*, **22,** 255–260

Van Aylea, O. E. (1936) The ostium maxillare. Anatomic study of its surgical accessibility. *Archives of Otolaryngology*, **24,** 553–569

Wehrbein, H., Bauer, W., Wessing, G. and Diedrich, P. (1990) Der einflub des Kieferhohlenbodens auf die orthodontische Zahnbewegung. *Fortschritte Kieferorthopadie*, **51,** 345–351

Williams, P. L., Warwick, R., Dyson, M. and Bannister, L. H. (eds) (1989) *Gray's Anatomy*, 37th edn, Churchill Livingstone, Edinburgh

Chapter 2

Histology, physiology and pathophysiology

Histology of mucoperiosteum

The respiratory mucosa lining the maxillary sinus is continuous with that of the nose and the other paranasal sinuses through their ostia. It is a mucoperiosteum consisting of a single layer of pseudostratified, ciliated columnar epithelium containing mucus-secreting goblet cells; it rests on a thin lamina propria of loose connective tissue and elastic fibrils which is continuous with the underlying periosteum. It is frequently raised into a series of folds and ridges but is easily stripped from the underlying bone in surgical procedures.

Healthy antral mucosa is thicker than that of the other paranasal sinuses (Strachan, 1987) but thinner than nasal mucosa, being less than 1 mm thick. It is less vascular than the nasal mucosa and, when viewed through a fibreoptic antroscope (Pogrel, 1985), it looks pale pink with many small blood vessels traversing it.

The maxillary sinus epithelium is similar to that in the nose, trachea and bronchi, mastoids, middle ear and auditory tubes – hence the term respiratory epithelium. Each epithelial cell has about 200 cilia which project from its free surface and beat at a frequency of about 10–20 Hz at body temperature. With scanning electron microscopy, Halama *et al.* (1990) found a high density of ciliated epithelial cells in the maxillary sinus mucosa, except near the ostium where the density was decreased by half. On the other hand, the highest density of goblet cells in the epithelium of the maxillary sinus was found near the ostium but was still lower than in the nasal epithelium.

Regeneration

The maxillary sinus mucosa has a high regenerative capacity and will return to normal once an external cause of infection (for example, in the anterior ethmoidal sinus, or a periapical abscess discharging into the sinus) has been treated (Stammberger, 1989).

Normal functioning ciliated epithelium can regenerate after operative removal of the complete lining of the maxillary sinus. This epithelial regeneration occurs mainly by ingrowth from the margins of the operative opening into the sinus but also, to a lesser extent, from islands of mucosa left behind.

The maxillary sinus lamina propria is much thinner than that of the nasal mucosa (Figure 2.1). It contains fewer mucous and seromucous glands, and very few of the serous glands that are copious throughout the nose. The serous glands are important for humidification of inspired air and contribute to the maintenance

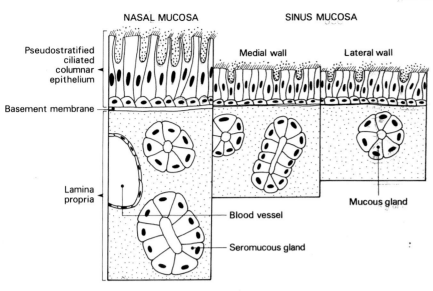

NASAL MUCOSA

SINUS MUCOSA

Pseudostratified
ciliated
columnar
epithelium

Medial wall

Lateral wall

Basement membrane

Lamina
propria

Mucous gland

Blood vessel

Seromucous gland

Figure 2.1 A diagrammatic comparison of nasal and sinus mucosa After Strachan (1987)

of the serous periciliary layer of the mucous blanket. The medial wall of the maxillary sinus has a lamina propria that is thicker and richer in seromucous glands than its lateral wall.

Cilia are cylindrical in shape and consist of an outer membrane surrounding nine pairs of peripheral microtubules and two central microtubules (Figure 2.2). Central and peripheral microtubules are connected by radiating secondary fibres. The central microtubules are separate from each other, each being termed a singlet. Each peripheral doublet has an A microtubule with a complete wall and a B microtubule which shares a quarter of the wall of the A microtubule.

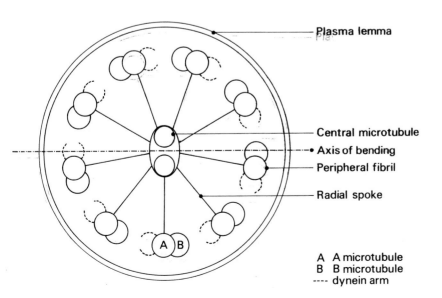

Plasma lemma

Central microtubule

Axis of bending

Peripheral fibril

Radial spoke

A A microtubule
B B microtubule
---- dynein arm

Figure 2.2 Transverse section of a cilium

Microtubules consist of tubulin dimers in a side-by-side arrangement. The A microtubule has two dynein arms projecting from it. Dynein arms are rich in adenosine triphosphatase activity and in the presence of high concentrations of calcium make temporary bridges with adjacent B microtubules. Addition of adenosine triphosphate produces a sliding movement of the bridge and, with a succession of temporary bridges and sliding movements, the dynein arms 'walk' along the B microtubules. The cilium is bent along a plane perpendicular to the axis through the central doublet.

Cilia undergo a regular and synchronous undulating movement, like a dancing effect. The effective stroke is a rapid forward movement with the cilium in a rigid state. It is followed by the slower recovery stroke, during which the cilium is flexible. Ciliary propulsion of mucus is achieved by a work stroke with the tips of the cilia in the mucous layer, followed by a recovery stroke which occurs in the serous layer (Figure 2.3).

The epithelial cilia beat continuously and provide a ciliary-driven sticky escalator, moving at a rate of 6 mm/min, transporting mucus and any adherent particles to the ostium, through it into the nose, and then to the nasopharynx to be swallowed (Figure 2.4). The mucous blanket consists of a serous layer, the periciliary fluid, adjacent to the epithelial cells, and a viscous overlying surface layer. Preservation of the width of the serous layer is essential for the movement of the mucus. If the serous layer becomes dehydrated and narrowed the mucus clings to the goblet cells secreting it, and to the cilia, and the clearance mechanism is rendered ineffective. Majima *et al.* (1986) suggested that this may occur in patients with chronic sinusitis, even when the mucociliary beat and mucus constituents are normal, and that nebulization with saline may be beneficial.

Interference with the movement of the mucus by the cilia or blockage of the ostium predisposes the sinuses to inflammation, and particularly to secondary bacterial infection.

Figure 2.3 Diagram of ciliary beat pattern. From Drake-Lee (1987)

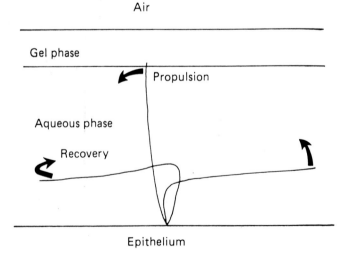

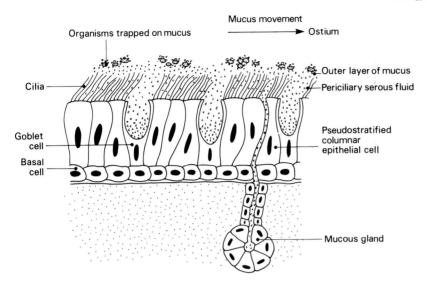

Figure 2.4 Mucus production and mucociliary transport

Physiology

The function of the maxillary sinuses is unknown. They may be products of the unusual growth patterns of the maxillae (Williams *et al.*, 1989).

As they are contiguous with the nose, they may help to add resonance to the voice, to smell, clean, warm and humidify inspired air, and modify expired air (Blanton and Biggs, 1969). Most authors are sceptical and consider that the sinuses contribute little except mucus production and, like the appendix, are notable only when diseased.

Reduction of weight of the facial skeleton

Having maxillary sinuses filled with air rather than cancellous bone lightens the face by approximately the weight of a pair of spectacles. Elephants have extensive sinuses which may reduce the weight of the skull, but their neck muscles are capable of supporting the weight of their large tusks and a man sitting on their head (McMinn, 1990).

Phonetic resonance and auditory feedback

The sinuses may act as a resonating box for the singing voice. The sinuses also affect the conductance of the voice to one's own ear. Pathological obliteration of one sinus was appreciated as asymmetrical resonance by a patient being trained in voice production (see Chapter 7). Joan Sutherland, the Australian operatic soprano found that after surgery for sinusitis, the resonance of her voice did not feel or sound the same (*Omnibus*, 1991). However, the subject is controversial. Drake-Lee (1987) agrees that the sinuses may aid auditory feedback but states that they do not modify the voice.

Negus (1958) studied other mammals and found no correlation between the presence of paranasal sinuses and the power of the voice; the giraffe has enormous frontal air spaces but is usually silent.

Insulation

The temperature of the inspired air can vary from $-50°C$ to $50°C$. The rich nasal arterial countercurrent on the turbinates warms the inspired air and may absorb heat from the expired air but 10% of body heat loss still occurs through the nose. The sinuses may insulate the orbits from intranasal temperature variations.

Air conditioning

As the posterior lateral nasal branches of the sphenopalatine artery run forwards over the turbinates they send branches which run towards the surface of the mucosa, where they divide into arterioles. Some of these arteries supply a subepithelial network of capillaries and others supply the glands and submucosal tissues. Arteriovenous anastomoses are common and are part of a complex system of pseudoerectile tissue which functions as a heat exchanger, maintaining an even and tolerable temperature and humidifying the inspired air. There is no anatomical evidence of such a mechanism in the sinus mucosa.

The maxillary sinuses do contain some serous glands whose watery secretion evaporates to humidify the contained air. The paranasal sinuses may act as supplementary chambers, helping the nose to warm, humidify and filter inspired air. Normal respiratory excursions are accompanied by fluctuations in intranasal and intra-antral pressure that are of equal magnitude and practically simultaneous. According to Drettner (1980), 90% exchange of the air in the maxillary sinus takes about 5 minutes during quiet nasal breathing and 10 minutes during oral breathing.

Water conservation

Moisture is critical to ciliary function. Dehydration for a few minutes will deplete the mucous blanket, stop ciliary beating and cause ciliary degeneration. Warm air can hold more moisture than cool air. Although they lack pseudoerectile tissue, the sinuses may act as accessory heat exchangers, warming inspired air to increase its moisture content, then cooling expired air to decrease its water content.

As camels inhabit an extremely dry environment with very large diurnal temperature changes, the heat exchanger role of their paranasal sinuses may have an important role in conserving their body water.

Filtration

Slavin (1988) suggested that particulate matter which escaped filtration by the nose may be trapped on the mucous blanket of the sinuses.

Olfaction

Pneumatization may have evolved to increase the area of olfactory mucosa, thereby improving the sense of smell (Negus, 1958). A scent may persist within the sinuses for some time and be used as a reference for any new odours experienced. In keen-scented carnivores, portions of the sphenoidal and frontal sinuses may be occupied by ethmoturbinal bodies and serve as extensions of the olfactory area (Weiss, 1988). Moore (1981) argues that the range of animals displaying this phenomenon, and the increase in olfactory epithelium, is too limited to make this explanation acceptable. In any case, maxillary sinuses in man do not contain olfactory epithelium.

Dead space

The masticatory stress in the maxilla is transmitted from the alveolar processes to the skull by three vertical buttresses whose size and shape is dictated by their function (Scott and Symons, 1974); the maxillary sinuses are simply the dead space in between. The sinuses may have evolved incidentally to the downward and forward growth of the face and the eruption of the teeth (Proetz, 1953) and persist in areas where there is no functional stimulus to bone formation.

Pathophysiology

While the function of the paranasal sinuses may be unknown, there has been considerable study of the various pathophysiological processes which are of clinical significance. These are: gas exchange of the maxillary sinus mucosa, patency of the ostium, blood flow, mucus production and mucociliary transport, and pressure changes in flying and diving.

Gas Exchange of the maxillary sinus mucosa

Far more oxygen is metabolized and consumed in mucociliary activity by the maxillary sinus mucosa than can be absorbed from the blood. Gas exchange is perfusion limited, not diffusion limited, and additional oxygen is absorbed from the air within the sinus (Drettner, 1980).

Mucosal oxygen consumption is normally in a steady state with exchange of oxygen through the antronasal duct, the functional bore of which determines the oxygen content of the air in the sinus. The usual diameter of 2.5 mm (5 mm^2 bore) or larger is required to maintain a normal oxygen tension (Po_2) of 116 mmHg, but below this diameter Po_2 is reduced, and falls to about 88 mmHg if the ostium is occluded. Sinusitis is more likely to occur in sinuses with small ostia and lower oxygen content (Aust and Drettner, 1974) (Figure 2.5). If gas exchange with air through the antronasal duct is impeded, as in maxillary sinusitis, a relatively anaerobic environment results and favours the growth of pathogenic bacteria.

The decrease in oxygen content of the air in the maxillary sinus after blockage of the antronasal duct causes increased capillary permeability and a transudate. This is followed by glandular metaplasia, an increase in numbers of goblet cells

Figure 2.5 The critical range of ostium size. Reduction from the normal bore of 5 mm² to complete occlusion is accompanied by a fall in Po_2 to 88 mmHg. If infection supervenes there is a further reduction in Po_2 within the sinus

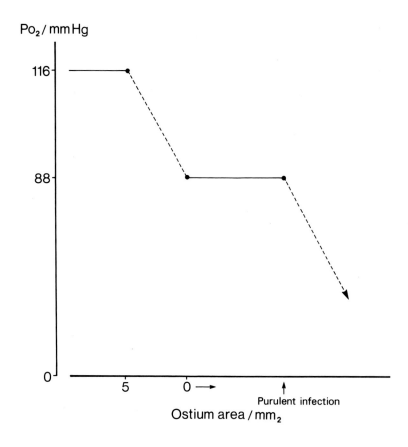

and a consequent increase in mucous secretion into the cavity. The hyperplastic mucosa eventually becomes oedematous and polypoidal and mucosal thickening is visible on a radiograph (Maran and Kerr, 1990) (See Figures 3.13, 3.16 (a)).

Patency of the antronasal duct

The maxillary sinus ostium leads into a 6 mm long curving canal (Grant, 1983), the whole being termed the antronasal duct. Antronasal duct patency is a prerequisite for the efficient aeration and clearance of secretions required to maintain a healthy maxillary sinus (Rohr and Spector, 1984). Aust, Drettner and Hemmingsson (1976) showed that the time to eliminate contrast medium from the maxillary sinus was inversely proportional to the size of the ostium. For optimum function the bore should be at least 5 mm², which is provided by a diameter of 2.5 mm. Although the mucociliary transport system in the sinus has been shown to function in the presence of pus (Toremalm, Merke and Reimer, 1975), if the ostium or channel becomes obstructed this transport of secretions is unavailing. The diameter of the lumen is variable, not only because the

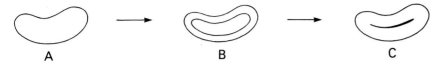

Figure 2.6 Diagram showing the effect of increasing thickness of the mucosal lining of the antronasal duct from A (no swelling), through B (1 mm swelling) to C (2 mm swelling) and complete blockage

anatomical opening varies in size but also because pathological processes may vary the thickness of the mucosa lining it. Like any other mucosa, that which lines the ostium or antronasal duct becomes swollen and engorged when acutely inflamed. The swollen sinus mucosa encroaches on the lumen concentrically so that the effect of even a modest increase in thickness is multiplied exponentially (Figure 2.6).

Nasal mucosal oedema also interferes with drainage of the sinus by encroaching on the ethmoidal infundibulum, through which the antronasal duct passes. Thus, coryza and its infective sequelae, vasomotor rhinitis and seasonal allergy, can compromise the patency of the antronasal duct.

The functional bore of the ostium may also be reduced by a plug of mucus, a polyp or, more rarely, a neoplasm, and is decreased by reclining from a sitting to a lying position (Drettner, 1980). Blockage of the antronasal duct may result from nasal septal deviation following injury, congenital defect or lateral displacement of the middle concha. Impaired antronasal communication predisposes to sinus barotrauma by preventing movement of air to equalize nasal and sinus pressure.

Because their nasal openings are above and in close proximity to the antronasal duct, pus from the frontal, anterior and middle ethmoid sinuses can readily drain into the maxillary sinuses. For this reason restoration of health of the ethmoid sinuses, in particular, is essential to the cure of maxillary sinusitis.

Sympathomimetic preparations such as ephedrine exert their effect by vasoconstriction and consequent reduction in bulk of the swollen mucosa. Xylometazoline has a more potent vasoconstrictor effect but may also reduce mucociliary function (Cervin *et al.*, 1988). In practice either preparation is effective.

Mucus production and mucociliary transport

Because the ostium is very close to the roof of the sinus, it is situated unfavourably for gravitational drainage when the head is erect (see Figure 1.2). Clearance of sinus secretions is therefore dependent on active transport by the mucociliary system.

Mucus is 95% water and contains small quantities of sialic acid, neutral polysaccharides, albumin, immunoglobulin A and lysosyme, as well as epithelial cells and phagocytes. Its presence as a surface layer decreases water loss, provides a mechanical barrier between the mucosa and atmospheric irritants, and traps particulate matter.

In Young's syndrome, which consists of sinusitis, obstructive azoospermia, and bronchiectasis or bronchitis (Young, 1970), the sinus and respiratory secretions are very viscous and, though the cilia are normal, mucociliary transport is decreased at all sites. The same problem arises in cystic fibrosis (mucoviscoidosis) where mucus production is congenitally abnormal.

The time for a saccharin particle placed on the superior surface of the inferior turbinate to reach the oropharynx and be appreciated as a sweet taste provides a measure of the fastest rate of nasal mucus transport (Andersen *et al.*, 1974). The mean flow rate is 6 mm/min but with a wide variation from 1 mm/min to over 20 mm/min. The test does not provide specific information regarding mucociliary transport within the antrum, but it may be assumed that defective nasal transport is likely to be reflected in reduced sinus mucosal function.

Mucociliary transport is necessary to prevent collection of fluid in the maxillary sinus and secondary infection. Ciliary propulsion begins in the base of the sinus, and cilia continue to beat towards the natural ostium even after nasal antrostomy in the inferior meatus. Inflammation, injury, adrenaline, corticosteroids, tobacco smoke, structural abnormalities of the cilia, and a combination of low partial pressure of oxygen in the sinus air and arterial blood will all decrease mucociliary transport. Temperatures above 45°C or below 10°C, application of 10% cocaine hydrochloride or desiccation will stop ciliary movement, and upper respiratory tract infection may result in sloughing of the epithelial cells.

Cilia are active even in the presence of pus (Toremalm, Merke and Reimer, 1975), although their number is reduced and they beat more slowly than normal. This is apparently due to the effect of bacterial toxins and elastase released from neutrophils (Wilson *et al.*, 1986). They even continue to be active for a short time after death.

Primary ciliary dyskinesia is an inherited defect in ciliary mobility affecting all cilia throughout the body. Kartagener's syndrome, which is due to the absence of dynein arms on the A subfibrils, consists, in addition to sinusitis, of bronchitis, situs inversus, and male infertility due to decreased sperm motility or decreased female fertility due to impaired transport of the ovum through the oviduct (Kartagener, 1933). Other ciliary defects are caused by transposition of microtubules and the absence of radial spokes.

The virus causing the common cold decreases mucus clearance for 1 – 2 weeks, which may help explain why a bacterial sinusitis can follow. Bacterial sinusitis does not inhibit ciliary function unless it causes epithelial necrosis. In sinusitis secondary to dental abscess, patches of ciliated columnar cells persist but most are eroded or converted to squamous epithelium.

Other clearance mechanisms

The negative air pressure during inspiration assists ciliary clearance from the maxillary sinus by the Venturi principle, whereby the rapid passage of air across the opening of the sinus creates a negative pressure and a suction effect. Snell (1986) states that drainage of mucus is also achieved by the syphon action created during blowing the nose.

Sneezing may also aid clearance by enhancing the Venturi effect. Irritation of the nasal mucosa causes sneezing when afferent stimuli in the maxillary nerve pass via the trigeminal ganglion to the brain, and through a reticulospinal relay to the phrenic nucleus, and hence to motor cells in the spinal cord which supply the intercostal and other respiratory muscles. Spontaneous exfoliation of roots which had been displaced into the antrum has occurred in this way (Killey and Kay, 1964). Sneezing has also been implicated in the pathogenesis of pneumocele of the maxillary antrum (Noyek *et al.*, 1977).

Flying and diving

Antral barotrauma occurs only if the antronasal duct is blocked. The effect is less common but more dramatic in diving than in flying.

The further from the earth's core, the lower is the ambient pressure of the surrounding air or water. Atmospheric pressure halves every 5500 metres ascended from sea level and, because of this exponential relationship, the change in pressure with height is greater at low altitudes (Figure 2.7). Pressurizing an aircraft's cabin maintains the higher pressures which exist at ground or low levels but still in the range where a small change in altitude produces a large change in pressure, so predisposing to barotrauma. It is therefore important for passenger comfort that a starting altitude and rate of pressurization and decompression are selected which allow time for adaptation.

In water, the variation in pressure with the depth is relatively far greater, increasing by 1 atmosphere for every 10 metres descended (Figure 2.8). Boyle's law states that the pressure (*P*) and volume (*V*) of a given mass of gas in an elastic container are inversely proportional (*PV* = constant), so that pressure changes will affect the volume of the mass of air in the sinuses. Expansion occurs on ascent, and contraction on descent.

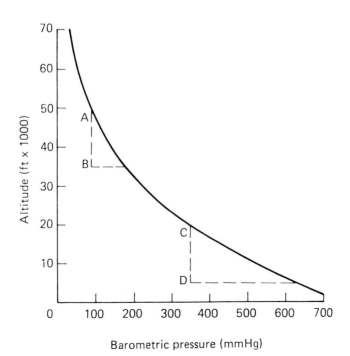

Figure 2.7 Relationship between altitude and barometric pressure in flight. For any given rate of descent, the rate of pressure change increases as the altitude is reduced. A descent of 15 000 ft (4570 m) is shown at AB and CD: in AB the pressure change is 91 mmHg (12.1 kPa) and in CD it is 283 mmHg (37.6 kPa). From Benson and King (1987)

Figure 2.8 Pressure–volume graph showing that the maximum change occurs during the first 10 m of a dive. From Benson and King (1987)

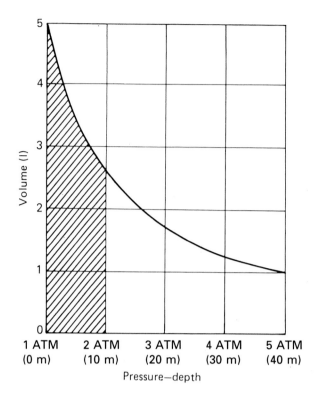

If the ostium is patent, air will pass out of it during ascent and back in during descent. Obstruction of the maxillary sinus's only opening precludes equalization of air pressure in the sinus with that of the surroundings. If the obstruction is valvular, such as occurs when a polyp is sucked over the ostium, relief may be obtained by attempted inspiration or expiration against closed anterior nares. The fontanelles may permit some expansion of the volume of the sinus during ascent or decrease in volume during descent, but with continued change in ambient pressure sinus barotrauma will occur. Severe pain develops suddenly in the cheeks shortly after pressure change, and epistaxis and rhinorrhoea may follow. During descent the absolute blood pressure increases and, because the air pressure in the obstructed sinus remains low, the sinus mucosa becomes engorged. If the pressure difference is large and prolonged, mucosal blood vessels may rupture, producing a subepithelial haematoma or haemorrhage.

The differential diagnosis of antral barotrauma includes dental barotrauma, which is more common, affecting one in five American fighter pilots (Ashley, 1977). Gas formed during pulpal autolysis expands on ascent, forcing infected material through the apex and causing severe pain, or, more commonly, pulpitis produces pain on ascent at about 2000 metres. Radiographs may be helpful in determining the cause and effect of the barotrauma.

Immediate treatment of sinus barotrauma involves analgesia, antihistamines and nasal decongestants to relieve the pain and unblock the ostium. Recurrence should then be prevented by removal of any tissue which may block the ostium or by antrostomy.

References

Andersen, I., Camner, P., Jensen, P. L. Philipson, K. and Proctor, D. F. (1974) Nasal clearance in monozygotic twins. *American Review of Respiratory Disorders*, **110**, 301–305

Ashley, K. F. (1977) Aerodontalgia – pain felt in the teeth during flight. *Medical and Dental Newsletter*, **26**, 15–17, Ministry of Defence (RAF), London

Aust, R. and Drettner, B. (1974) Oxygen tension in the human maxillary sinus under normal and pathological conditions. *Acta Oto-laryngologica (Stockholm)*, **78**, 264–269

Aust, R., Drettner, B. and Hemmingsson, A. (1976) Elimination of contrast medium from the maxillary sinus. *Acta Oto-laryngologica (Stockholm)*, **81**, 468–474

Benson, A. J. and King, P. F. (1987) Pathophysiology of the ears and nasal sinus in flying and diving. In *Scott-Brown's Otolaryngology*, Vol. 1, 5th edn (ed. D. Wright), Butterworth–Heinemann, Oxford, chap. 7

Blanton, P. L. and Biggs, N. L. (1969) Eighteen hundred years of controversy: the paranasal sinuses. *American Journal of Anatomy*, **124**, 135–148

Cervin, A., Bende, M., Lindberg, S., Mercke, U. and Olsson, P. (1988) Relation between blood flow and mucociliary activity in the rabbit maxillary sinus. *Acta Otolaryngologica (Stockholm)*, **105**, 350–356

Drake-Lee, A. B. (1987) Physiology of the nose and paranasal sinuses. In *Scott-Brown's Otolaryngology*, Vol. 1, 5th edn (ed. D. Wright), Butterworth-Heinemann, Oxford, Chap. 6

Drettner, B. (1980) Pathophysiology of paranasal sinuses with clinical implications. *Clinical Otolaryngology*, **5**, 277–284

Grant, J. C. B. (1983) *Grant's Atlas of Anatomy*, 8th edn, Williams and Wilkins, Baltimore

Halama, A. R., Decreton, S., Bijloos, J. M. and Clement, P. A. (1990) Density of epithelial cells in the normal human nose and the paranasal sinus mucosa. A scanning electron microscopic study. *Rhinology*, **28**, 25–32

Kartagener, M. (1933) Zum pathogenese der bronkiektasien bei situs viscerum inversus. *Beitrage zur Klinik und Erforschung der Tuberkulose und der lungen Krantheiten*, **83**, 489–501

Killey, H. C. and Kay, L. W. (1964) Possible sequelae when a tooth or root is dislodged into the maxillary sinus. *British Dental Journal*, **116**, 73–77

McMinn, R. M. H. (ed.) (1990) *Last's Anatomy Regional and Applied*, 8th edn, Churchill Livingstone, Edinburgh, p. 473

Majima, Y., Sakakura, Y., Matsubara, T. and Miyoshi, Y. (1986) Possible mechanisms of reduction of nasal mucociliary clearance in chronic sinusitis. *Clinical Otolaryngology*, **11**, 55–60

Maran, A. G. D. and Kerr, A. I. G. (1990) What's new in surgery: otolaryngology. *Journal of the Royal College of Surgeons of Edinburgh*, **35**, 140–143

Moore, W. J. (1981) *In Biological Structure and Function*, (eds Harrison and McMinn), 8. *The Mammalian Skull*, Cambridge University Press, Cambridge, pp. 277–279

Negus, V. (1958) *The Comparative Anatomy and Physiology of the Nose and Paranasal Sinuses*, E. and S. Livingstone, Edinburgh, pp. 320–327

Noyek, A. M., Zizmor, J., Morrison, M. D., Vines, F. S. and Shaffer, K. (1977) The radiologic diagnosis of pneumocele of the maxillary sinus. *Journal of Otolaryngology. Supplement*, **3**, 17–21

Omnibus, BBC1 television programme, 11th July 1991

Pogrel, M. A. (1985) Fiberoptic antroscopy. *Journal of Oral and Maxillofacial Surgery*, **43**, 139–142

Proetz, A. W. (1953) *Applied Physiology of the Nose*, 2nd edn, Mosby, St Louis

Rohr, A. S. and Spector, S. L. (1984) Paranasal sinus anatomy and pathophysiology. *Clinical Review of Allergy*, **2,(1B)** 387–395

Scott, J. H. and Symons, N. B. B. (1974) *Introduction to Dental Anatomy*, 7th edn, Churchill Livingstone, Edinburgh

Slavin, R. G. (1988) Sinusitis in adults (symposium). *Journal of Allergy and Clinical Immunology*, **81**, 1028–1032

Snell, R. S. (1986) *Clinical Anatomy for Medical Students*, 3rd edn, Little, Brown, Boston

Stammberger, H. (1959) *Functional Endoscopic Nasal and Paranasal Sinus Surgery – The Messerklinger Technique (MT)*, Braun-Druck, Tuttlingen, pp. 1, 34

Strachan, D. S. (1987) Nasal cavity, paranasal sinuses, and tonsils. In *Oral Development and Histology*, Williams and Wilkins, Baltimore, pp. 222–230.

Toremalm, N. G., Merke, U. and Reimer, A. (1975) The mucociliary activity of the upper respiratory tract. *Rhinology*, **13**, 113–120

Weiss, L. (1988) *Cell and Tissue Biology. A Textbook of Histology*, 6th edn, Urban and Schwarzenberg, Munich, pp. 753–754

Williams, P. L., Warwick, R., Dyson, M., and Bannister, L. (eds) (1989) *Gray's Anatomy*, 37th edn, Churchill Livingstone, Edinburgh

Wilson, R., Sykes, D. A., Currie, D. and Cole, P. J. (1986) Beat frequency of cilia from sites of purulent infection. *Thorax*, **41**, 453–458

Young, D. (1970) Surgical treatment of male infertility. *Journal of Reproduction and Fertility*, **23**, 541–542

Chapter 3

Examination and investigation of the maxillary sinus

Clinical examination

Examination is generally preceded by the discussion and recording of the presenting complaint and its history, and the patient's general medical history.

The middle third of the face should be inspected for the presence of asymmetry, deformity, swelling, erythema, ecchymosis or haematoma. Epiphora, nasal obstruction, epistaxis or other discharge or odour from the nostril should be noted. In the absence of traumatic injury, paraesthesia of the infraorbital nerve is a potentially sinister sign. Examination should also include palpation of the facial wall of the sinus above the premolars, where the bone is thinnest, either through the soft tissues of the cheek, or more directly intraorally. Tenderness may be elicited in acute sinusitis, and swellings or fracture lines defined. Crepitus is indicative of surgical emphysema, which occurs when a mucosal tear is associated with a fracture of the sinus wall and air escapes into the subcutaneous tissues. Trismus may result from extension of an antral tumour to involve the pterygoid muscles.

Intraoral examination should be performed, looking for alveolar ulceration, expansion, tenderness, or paraesthesia of the upper molar and premolar region. Teeth should be tested for mobility, and dentures for retention and stability, as changes may be a sign of extension of a sinus tumour into the alveolus. Palatal ulceration should be biopsied if there is no obvious cause and it does not heal within 1 week.

The eyes should be examined for proptosis, upward displacement of the globe, seen as inequality of the pupillary level in forward gaze, or restriction of movement producing diplopia, especially on upward or on upward and lateral gaze.

The frontal and ethmoid sinuses should also be examined because disease of these structures frequently affects the antrum. The anterior ethmoid air cells can be palpated through the lamina papyracea of the medial wall of the orbit, and the frontal sinus by pressing upwards with the finger pulp from the superomedial angle of the orbit. Direct percussion of the anterior wall of the frontal sinus is carried out with the middle finger above the medial limit of the eyebrow. Cervical lymph nodes should be palpated.

Rhinoscopy

A nasal speculum and headlight or mirror are necessary for proper examination of the nasal passages. The technique of anterior rhinoscopy is well explained by

Marshall and Attia (1987). A topical vasoconstrictor may decrease the size of a large inferior turbinate which obstructs the view of the middle turbinate and middle meatus. Bull (1987) claims that, with the middle meatus exposed, the hiatus semilunaris and bulla ethmoidalis are seen anteriorly and it is possible to cannulate or probe the ostium more posteriorly. On the other hand, Kennedy *et al.* (1985) state that anterior rhinoscopy reveals little of the middle meatal cleft and nothing of the infundibular opening and maxillary sinus orifice. Pus may be seen in the middle meatus but it is difficult to determine its origin. It is important to realize that if a probe is passed anterior to the ostium it will pass through the thin lamina papyracea of the medial wall of the orbit.

Under local or general anaesthesia, and after in-fracturing and lifting of the turbinates to expose the inferior and middle meatuses, a longer bladed speculum is used to permit visualization of the middle and posterior thirds of the nasal cavities.

Posterior rhinoscopy using a nasopharyngeal mirror is necessary for visualization of the posterior aspects of all conchae.

Nasendoscopy

Under outpatient local anaesthesia the nasal opening of the maxillary sinus in the middle meatus may be examined more thoroughly using a narrow fibreoptic endoscope (Bull, 1987). This is particularly important because sinus disease usually starts in the middle meatus. A view of the superior meatus and a better view of the inferior meatus are also obtained.

Transillumination

Transillumination of the maxillary sinuses is simply performed in a darkened room by insertion of an electrically safe bright light into the mouth (with the lips closed) after removal of any maxillary prosthesis. A difference in luminosity between the two sinuses, seen best at the medial third of the infraorbital rim, indicates the presence of unilateral disease. A large cyst filled with clear fluid will be opaque on radiographs but brilliantly clear on transillumination (Mackay and Cole, 1987). Good transillumination indicates air in the sinuses, whereas failure of transillumination indicates the presence of pus, a solid lesion or mucosal thickening. A finding between these two extremes is rather difficult to interpret.

Transillumination is rarely performed nowadays as sophisticated methods of examination are more revealing.

Bacteriology and cytology

Proof puncture of the antrum is usually performed through the inferior meatus to confirm radiological appearances. Following topical vasoconstriction with 1:1000 adrenaline and analgesia with 10% cocaine spray, then solution, a trocar and cannula is passed under the attachment of the inferior turbinate up to the genu where it will naturally come to rest. The body of the trocar is held in the palm of the hand with the index finger running along its shaft to provide control

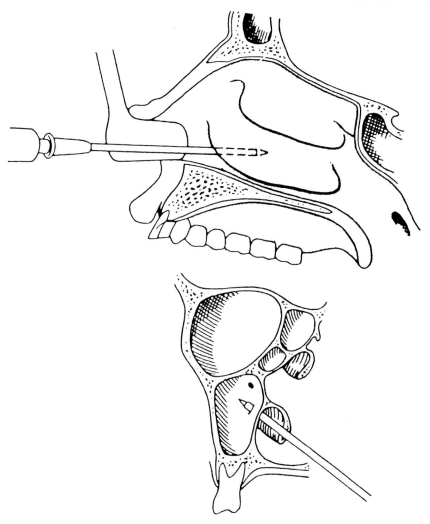

Figure 3.1 Line of introduction of trochar and cannula into the maxillary sinus. From Lund (1987)

and a 'stop'. It is directed towards the tragus of the ipsilateral ear while the patient's head is held still (Figure 3.1). Moderate pressure with a rotary movement will lead to perforation of the thinnest part of the lateral inferior meatal wall, which is just behind the lacrimal duct orifice. The trocar and cannula is advanced to the lateral sinus wall, then withdrawn several millimetres before the trocar is removed. An aspirate is withdrawn into an empty syringe and sent for bacteriological and cytological examination (Lund, 1987).

Fibreoptic antroscopy

Using this procedure, sinuses unresponsive to treatment or any 'suspicious' areas seen radiographically can be examined by direct vision through an endoscope (Figures 3.2 and 3.3).

Figure 3.2 Nasendoscopy and antroscopy reveals hidden areas of the nasal cavity and maxillary antrum. From Croft (1987)

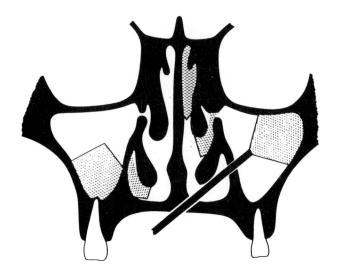

Figure 3.3 Antroscopic views. (a) Normal antral mucosa with one large patent ostium. (b) Hyperaemic mucosa with single obstructed ostium. (c) A large cyst within the antrum. (d) Thick mucus covering sinus floor. From Croft (1987)

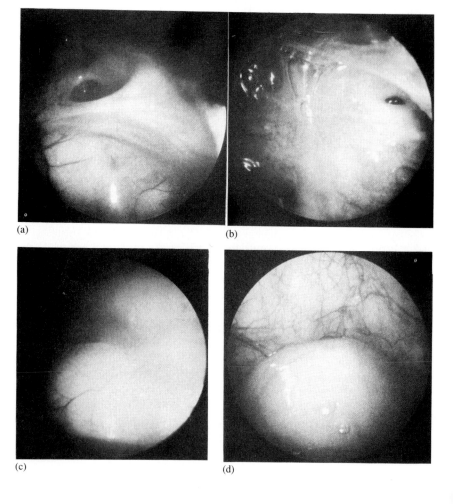

(a)

(b)

(c)

(d)

Antroscopy is the only definitive way to investigate the contents and lining of the maxillary sinus. It is quick, reasonably well tolerated, has a low associated morbidity, and can be performed as an outpatient procedure under local anaesthesia. Access to the antrum is either via an intranasal antrostomy or the canine fossa. The latter, Caldwell–Luc approach is more easily tolerated by patients and gives a better overall view of the antrum, and especially the ostium (Pogrel, 1985).

If the antrum is large and the facial wall is thin, no preliminary mucosal incision is required. The antrum is entered using a sharp trocar and cannula which can be pushed directly through the anaesthetized oral or nasal mucosa, bone and sinus mucosa into the antrum. The trocar is then removed and the endoscope is inserted along the cannula and attached to a light source. Bleeding is minimal when local anaesthesia is used, but if it does occur, suction can be accomplished and bleeding points clipped, though directing the artery forceps through the antroscopy is difficult. Alternatively, the forceps may be inserted into the antrum through a separate antrostomy and guided using the antroscope. Forceps with built-in suction may facilitate biopsy (I. Mackay, personal communication 1990).

Antroscopy is also said to be useful in identifying orbital blow-out fractures where clinical and radiological examination is inconclusive (Westjbal and Kreidler, 1977), although haemorrhage or blood clot may be a problem.

Nasal mucociliary clearance test (saccharine test)

This test was first described by Anderson *et al.* (1974) and is used to measure mucociliary function. A particle of saccharine is placed in the anterior part of the middle meatus. The subject swallows every 30 s and the time between placement and report of a sweet taste is the measure.

Nasal ciliary beat frequency

Strips of ciliated epithelium are brushed off the lateral aspect of the inferior turbinate and examined under a phase-contrast microscope. The number of effector strokes of the cilia per second is counted, the normal range being 12–15 Hz (Rutland, Griffin and Cole, 1982). Purulent infection decreases the ciliary beat frequency as a result of the release of neutrophil elastase (Smallman, Hill and Stockley, 1984) and bacterial toxins (Sykes *et al.*, 1986). Specimens are also examined to determine the percentage of immotile cilia.

Rhinomanometry

Active anterior rhinomanometry is the method of choice (Clement, 1984). It consists of the measurement of nasal air flow and pressure at the nostrils during respiration. The main clinical application is to determine whether a patient who complains of a nasal obstruction does indeed have one.

Radiology

A knowledge of normal radiological anatomy and any common variations is essential in order to distinguish pathological changes.

Both intraoral and extraoral radiographs are used to examine the maxillary sinuses. Extraoral views have the advantage of showing both sinuses on the same radiograph so that comparisons can be made. Gross changes are readily seen and a complete lesion is usually demonstrated on one radiograph. However, apart from dental panoramic views, extraoral radiography is seldom available in dental practice.

Intraoral views are taken with plain radiographic film, which has higher resolution than the intensifying screen–fast film combination used in extraoral radiography. An intraoral film therefore permits a more detailed examination of a specific area. As well as the sinus floor and surrounding alveolar bone, intraoral views demonstrate crown and root pathology, which may be helpful in accurately diagnosing disease of dental origin.

Intraoral radiographs

Both periapical and occlusal views may be useful. Despite its variable size and shape the maxillary sinus is usually seen on occlusal views and on periapical radiographs of the upper premolar and molar regions, unless it is very small. Its anterior limit lies in the region of the maxillary canine and it extends backwards to the tuberosity, which may be pneumatized.

One of the most constant anatomical radiographic features of the maxilla is the medial wall of the maxillary sinus which separates the nasal fossa from the sinus (Ennis and Batson, 1936; Ennis, 1937). In the canine region the opaque lines forming a Y shape are known as the 'Y of Ennis' (Figure 3.4). The anterior white

Figure 3.4 Original illustration showing the 'Y' of Ennis. See A and C from Ennis and Batson (1937)

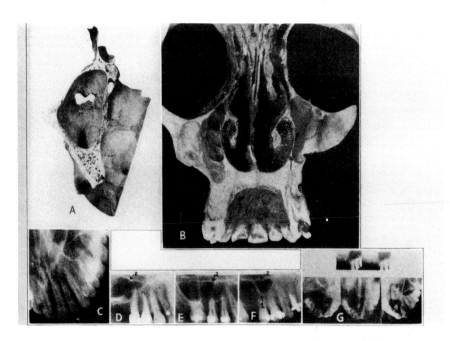

line represents the lower border of the lateral wall of the nasal fossa, which extends more anteriorly than the medial wall of the sinus. The posterior white lines are formed by the diverging facial and medial walls of the sinus. Knowledge of this Y is very important in differentiating pathology from normal anatomy on intraoral radiographs (Ennis, 1937).

Fine neurovascular channels in the bony lateral sinus walls and floor are represented by typical dark branching lines (Figure 3.5). Nutrient canals pass from them to the apices of the upper posterior teeth. As they are absent in cyst linings they are useful in determining whether or not a cyst is present. They should not be confused with fracture lines, which are less regular and smoothly curved. Other normal anatomical features include the zygomatic buttress which appears as a U- or V-shaped radiopacity in the region of the first and second molar roots (Figure 3.6). There may also be incomplete septa within the sinus, sometimes producing a loculated appearance similar to that of a cyst (Figure 3.7).

Both the upper anterior oblique occlusal and the upper lateral oblique occlusal views of the canine region show the anterior part of the hard palate and may reveal the full extent of a large cyst or other lesion in this region, which cannot be completely seen on a periapical film. Oblique occlusal views (Figure 3.8) may also be helpful in differentiating a cyst from the maxillary sinus or in locating a dislodged root, but will not demonstrate penetration of the antral wall.

A periapical view of the premolar region will show the floor of the maxillary sinus as a radiopaque line which may dip down between, cross or lie above the roots (Figure 3.9). The bone which separates the roots from the antral floor varies in thickness from zero to 2 cm, so the antrum may be too high to be seen on some periapical radiographs, particularly those taken with the long cone paralleling technique.

A radiograph of the molar region will reveal the extent of pneumatization of the maxillary tuberosity.

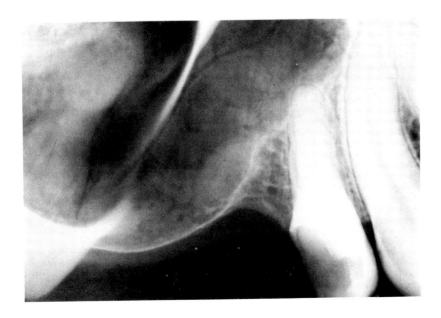

Figure 3.5 Periapical radiograph of 65┐ region showing neurovascular and nutrient canals in the walls of a very extensive antrum

Xeroradiography

X-rays are used to produce an image on specially charged selenium plates instead of radiographic film. This high contrast technique differentiates areas with subtle density differences so that bony trabeculae and tooth roots are clearly shown. However, the plates are more expensive than conventional radiographs and have been superseded by computed tomography (CT) for the investigation of the maxillary sinuses (Phelps, 1987b).

Figure 3.6 Periapical radiograph of U-shaped buttress and maxillary teeth

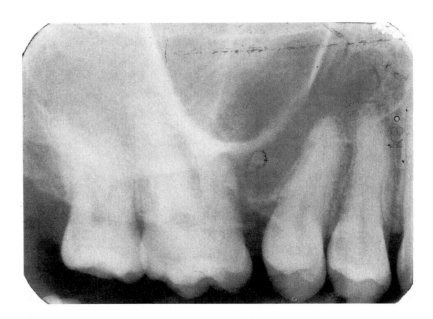

Figure 3.7 A clearly demarcated septum which has to be distinguished from a cyst wall

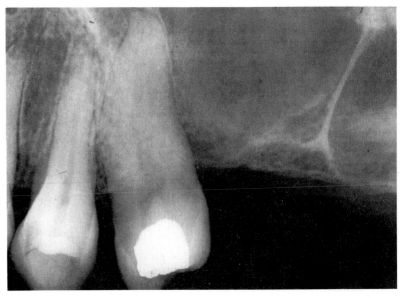

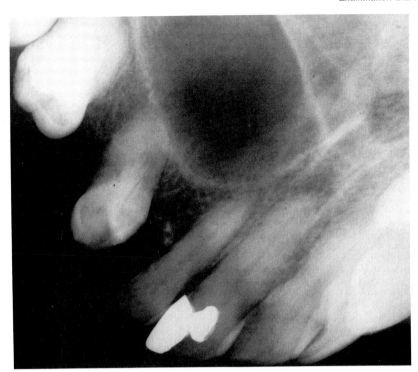

Figure 3.8 The maxillary sinus displayed on an oblique occlusal radiograph

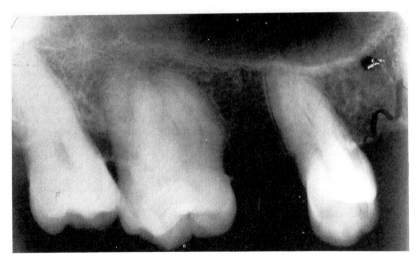

Figure 3.9 Periapical radiograph of the floor of the sinus in relation to the roots of the maxillary posterior teeth (same patient as Figure 3.8)

Extraoral radiographs

The two views in most widespread use are Waters' projection and the panoramic radiograph of the jaws (orthopantomograph). Ohba and Katayama (1976) compared them and found that cyst-like densities in the sinus were better detected on panoramic views, whereas cloudiness of the antrum and sclerotic change of adjacent bony structures were best demonstrated on the Waters' projection. The two techniques supplement one another and may be used together to obtain more accurate information.

Waters' view

This occipitomental radiograph was first described by Waters and Waldron (1915) and is the view most commonly used in hospital practice to examine the maxillary sinus (Figure 3.10). Nowadays this view is taken with the orbitomeatal line, which passes from the outer canthus of the eye to the centre of the external auditory meatus, at an angle of 45° to the film. The patient's chin rests on the cassette, the nose is approximately 1–1.5 cm from it and the central ray is at 90° to the film. It is preferable to take this view with the patient's head erect to demonstrate any fluid level within the sinus.

A clear view of the maxillary sinus, its medial and lateral walls, its roof and the inferior orbital rim is obtained. The roof of the sinus appears 1–3 mm below and parallel to the inferior orbital rim. Asymmetrical increase in this distance occurs in orbital blow-out fracture.

Overangled or underangled occipitomental radiographs give tangential views of the roof of the antrum, which may be useful in cases of facial trauma (Phelps, 1987).

The ethmomaxillary plate which separates the maxillary and ethmoid sinuses is destroyed in aggressive inflammatory or malignant disease. When viewing occipitomental radiographs, the canal for the posterior superior dental vessels and nerve, the infraorbital foramen and the zygomatic and alveolar recesses should be identified as normal sinus components. The infraorbital canal near the middle of the sinus roof and the canal for the posterior superior dental nerve and vessels on the lateral walls may mimic fractures.

The image of the zygomatic process may resemble mucosal thickening. Unerupted molars in the tuberosity region can simulate the air/fluid level of acute sinusitis but a panoramic radiograph or a lateral view will reveal the unerupted teeth. The superior orbital fissure, foramen rotundum, foramen ovale, the lateral border of the posterior ethmoid and sphenoid sinuses and the inferior extension of the temporal line are other external structures which may be superimposed on the antrum (Yanagisawa and Smith, 1976).

The temporal or innominate line, which represents the depths of the depression on the lateral surface of the greater wing of the sphenoid bone, is superimposed on the lateral aspect of the orbit. It is often projected inferiorly as the infratemporal extension over the superolateral part of the sinus, ending either in a straight line or turning medially. The posterior ethmoid air cells are superimposed on the superomedial part of the sinus. The superior orbital fissure is projected as a tear-shaped radiolucency passing from the inferior orbital rim inferomedially and crossing the medial wall of the sinus. The foramen rotundum, which is always lateral to the lower end of the superior orbital fissure, and the foramen ovale may simulate a cyst or bone erosion (Yanagisawa and Smith, 1976). A disadvantage of the Waters' view is that in the posteroinferior region the sinus is obscured by the petrous temporal bone or alveolus.

Other plain views of the antra

The anterior and posterior parts of the roof and the lateral walls of the antra are seen on the occipitofrontal (Caldwell) view. The submentovertical view clearly demonstrates the S-shaped antral line which represents the posterolateral walls of the maxillary sinuses. In lateral views the sinuses are superimposed, making it difficult to tell if the pathology is located on the left or the right. Posteroanterior and lateral views should no longer be used as sinus screening films (Southwood, 1990).

Lateral cephalograms (Figure 3.11) are taken with the Frankfort plane horizontal. This passes through orbitale, the lowest point in the floor of the left orbit, to porion, the highest point of each external auditory meatus. The zygomatic buttress, anterior and posterior boundaries of the medial wall of the antrum, and the anterior wall of the pterygoid process of the sphenoid bone are demonstrated. If lateral cephalograms are taken for orthognathic or orthodontic reasons the clinician should still examine the sinuses.

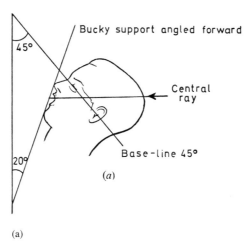

(a)

Figure 3.10 Waters' (occipitomental) view of the sinuses: (a) technique; (b) radiograph; (c) line drawing of (b). 1, Frontal sinuses; 2, nasal bones; 3, nasal process of maxilla; 4, nasal septum; 5, middle turbinate; 6, posterolateral wall of antrum; 7, antrum; 8, anterolateral wall of antrum; 9, inferior turbinate; 10, sphenoid sinus; 11, foramen ovale overlying alveolar recess of antrum; 12, soft tissue shadow cast by lips (dotted lines); 13, foramen rotundum; 14, infraorbital foramen; 15, zygoma; 16, superior orbital fissure; 17, innominate line; 18, lamina papyracea of ethmoid; 19, frontozygomatic suture; 20, soft tissue shadow cast by nares (dotted lines); 21, orbit; 22, ethmoid cells. From Phelps (1987)

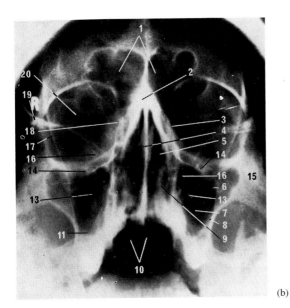

(b)

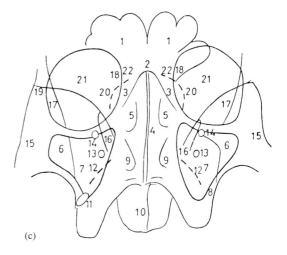

(c)

Figure 3.11 Lateral cephalogram
showing the two maxillary sinuses

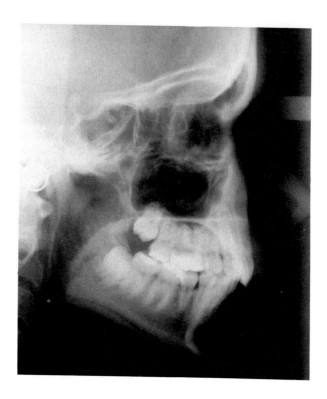

Figure 3.12 Panoramic radiograph
shows the maxillary sinuses as dark
areas above the upper posterior
tooth roots

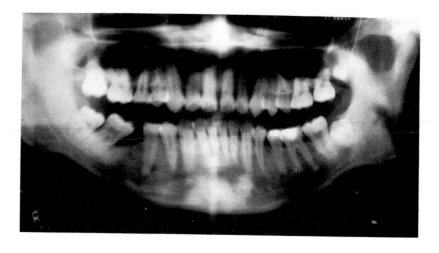

Panoramic radiograph of the jaws

Panoramic radiographs are obtained by synchronized rotation of the X-ray tube and film around the patient, producing a clear image of only a curved strip of tissue (Figure 3.12 and see Figure 1.12). The panoramic tomographic view is built up by consecutive single exposures of each vertical strip of film. The area recorded is a thick (2–3 cm) cut through the maxillary sinus in the same plane as the upper dental arch. The panoramic radiograph is therefore similar to a frontal view anteriorly and a lateral view posteriorly.

The narrow beam used causes minimal scatter which results in good contrast (Paukku *et al.*, 1983a). The average patient radiation dose to the bone marrow is low, being approximately equivalent to that of four bite-wings (White and Rose, 1979) or four periapical exposures.

While it is an excellent screening radiograph, a small lesion outside the plane of the cut will be missed.

Although the image quality is not as good as that of intraoral radiographs, a wide area is viewed in one exposure. The panoramic radiograph is better than the Waters' projection for demonstrating the antral floor (see Figure 1.12).

Flat plane tomography

This is the simplest version of the technique: a thin (1–2 mm), sharply-defined flat plane 'section' of the patient is displayed while structures anterior and posterior to the section are blurred. The effect is achieved by controlled movement of both the tube and the film around a single pivot which remains 'in focus'. The whole film is continuously exposed, resulting in a series of very faint images superimposed on each other. In the preselected flat plane, or tomographic 'cut', there is no relative movement of the tube and film and the image is sharp. A series of cuts is usually produced at different depths throughout the region of interest. These tomograms are of particular benefit in blow-out fractures of the orbital floor to locate the fracture site, and in establishing the extent of a tumour in the antrum.

Hypocycloidal or spiral tomography is preferable as fine bone detail can be demonstrated without streaking (Phelps, 1987). In larger hospitals, both have been superseded by CT.

Panoramic zonography

In this technique the rotation of the tube, rotation of the film and vertical movement of the carriage are controlled separately, permitting the programming of different cuts (Hallikainen and Paukku, 1990). The maxillary sinuses may be imaged in a cylindrical, concave, 14 or 28 mm cut with the patient in the reversed Waters' position. The soft tissue swelling and bony dislocation following blow-out fractures of the orbital floor are easily seen (see Figure 5.28), as is damage to the lateral wall of the sinus in middle-third or zygomatic complex fractures. Maxillary cysts encroaching on the sinus or mucus retention cysts arising within it will also be revealed. Thinner cuts may be taken if bony erosion is suspected in inflammatory or neoplastic disease. The reversed Waters' cuts of the maxillary sinus are diagnostically superior to plain radiographs and involve significantly lower radiation doses to the eye, thyroid and parotid (Paukku *et al.*, 1983b).

Figure 3.13 Coronal CT scan showing a healthy right maxillary sinus and some mucosal thickening in the lower lateral part of the left maxillary sinus

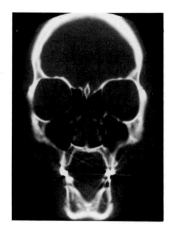

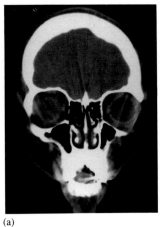

(a)

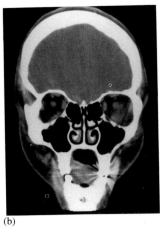

(b)

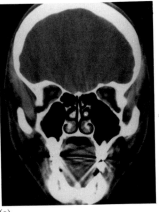

(c)

Figure 3.14 (a)–(c) Series of coronal CT scans of a healthy subject demonstrating the size, shape and relationship of the maxillary sinuses from anterior to posterior

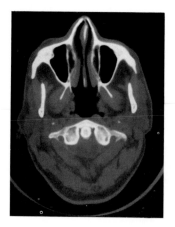

Figure 3.15 Axial CT scan showing the thickness of the mucosa lining the antra septum and turbinates

As the thickness of the cut for the lateral view is 12 cm it is very similar to an ordinary film and offers little advantage.

Computed tomography

Computer-aided production of images from X-rays was developed and introduced into clinical use by the British physicist Godfrey Hounsfield in 1972. As a result of this work, Dr Hounsfield and Professor A. M. Cormack were jointly awarded the Nobel prize for medicine in 1979.

Data collected during multidirectional X-ray scanning of the object are analysed by computer in a technique which is usually known as CT (computed tomography) scanning. The appearance of the tissues varies with the level and angle of the scan section, the most commonly used being the axial (tranverse) and coronal scans. By utilizing both axial and coronal scans, a three-dimensional image of both normal and abnormal structures can be obtained (Figures 3.13 and 3.14).

CT more clearly contrasts the air–soft tissue lining interface, and the mucosa–bone junction in the nose and sinuses (Figure 3.15a and b). Most importantly, it will reveal disease extending beyond the bony margins of the sinus into adjacent soft tissues (Phelps, 1987). Contrast enhancement is useful in demonstrating the start of soft tissue spread. CT is more sensitive than conventional tomography in the examination of the paranasal sinuses because it more consistently identifies thin spicules of bone.

It is important to be familiar with both hard and soft tissue anatomy when interpreting CT scans, as the involvement of surrounding tissues is determined by recognizing destruction and displacement of normal structures rather than by direct visualization of abnormal tissue.

CT scans taken after blow-out fractures of the medial wall, or particularly the floor of the orbit may show orbital contents displaced into the maxillary sinus (see Chapter 4). A CT scan of the brain may reveal intracranial lesions after maxillofacial trauma.

Axial scans are parallel to the orbital–meatal baseline, which forms an angle of 10° with the Frankfort plane. The axial view can be taken without having to place a very ill patient in awkward or potentially dangerous positions. Using data obtained from many thin slices the computer can reconstruct an indirect coronal view. Facial bones, paranasal sinuses, the skull base and the postnasal space are all clearly seen in axial sections. The posterolateral walls of the maxillary sinuses, together with the soft tissue structures of the infratemporal and pterygopalatine fossae, which are clearly demarcated, are areas difficult to demonstrate by any other technique (see Chapter 6). Extension of a tumour into the infratemporal fossa is clinically apparent only when trismus is present, by which stage invasion is extensive and treatment possibilities are restricted. The ability to detect tumour spread earlier is therefore of great potential advantage.

Coronal scans are valuable for assessing extension of paranasal sinus disease in palatal, orbital and nasal directions. True coronal scans are taken in the submentovertical position with the patient's neck extended, but may be difficult to obtain because of patient intolerance or machine limitations. Stammberger and Wolf (1988) suggest that coronal CTs should always be taken as they permit optimum visualization of the narrow compartments of the lateral nasal wall, including the key areas of the ethmoid infundibulum and the frontal recess.

Unfortunately, metal restorations or crowns may cause interference, especially on coronal CT scans (Figures 3.13 and 3.14b,c). Phelps (1987) suggests that this may be decreased by changing the angle of the gantry or the position of the patient's head. However, Stammberger and Wolf (1988) find that artefacts caused by metallic dental restorations do not interfere with the critical examination of the sinuses on direct coronal CT scans. Perez and Farman (1988) compared CT with periapical, occlusal, angled posterior and panoramic radiographic techniques in visualizing simulated maxillary sinus defects in dried human skulls. While CT was best, simple periapical films were equally effective in suitable areas.

The main disadvantage of CT is its cost. It is also not sensitive enough to predict precise tissue histopathology unless the lesion is very vascular or has undergone characteristic calcification.

Magnetic resonance imaging

Magnetic resonance imaging (MRI) is a newer diagnostic technique based upon work by Paul Lauterbur (Lauterbur, 1973). The major advantage is that no ionizing radiation is used and therefore it is free of the associated hazards.

A simple outline of the very complex physics underlying the production of images is as follows. Both intracellular and extracullular hydrogen ions are lined up parallel to its field by a very powerful external magnet. A pulse of radiowaves at a critical frequency (precessional) is absorbed by the hydrogen ions, which change their orientation by 90°, spin in the transverse plane and emit their own radiofrequency signal (Newhouse and Wiener, 1991). This signal is detected and used to create the image.

When the radiowaves stop, the time it takes the hydrogen ions to release energy and return to being parallel to the magnetic field depends on their chemical environment. Thus, hydrogen in water gives a different signal from hydrogen in fat. As the fat and water content of different normal and abnormal tissues vary, so does the signal they produce. T_1 and T_2 relaxation times are two measures of the energy absorbing and releasing characteristics. In a T_1 weighted image, fat gives a white bright high intensity signal and water a dark low intensity signal. The reverse occurs in T_2 weighting (Barrett, Poliakoff and Holder, 1990).

MRI is extremely sensitive in demonstrating maxillary sinus mucosal pathology due to the high signal intensity on T_2 weighted images of almost all soft tissue abnormalities, contrasted with the absence of signal from both the air within the sinus and the surrounding cortical bone (Moser *et al.*, 1991) (Figure 3.16). It is important to note that because the hydrogen ions in cortical bone are tightly bound they do not produce a signal. Thus, MRI will not demonstrate tumour infiltration of the bony walls of the maxillary sinus but, because of their surrounding layer of fat, the displacement or destruction of facial muscles is well demonstrated.

MRI is the most sensitive technique available for visualizing intracerebral pathology. While examining MRI brain scans, Moore *et al.* (1986) found that some incidental paranasal sinus pathology was clearly revealed. They suggested that the technique might be useful in the study of the nature and epidemiology of inflammatory sinus disease. However, Moser *et al.* (1991), who found 25% of

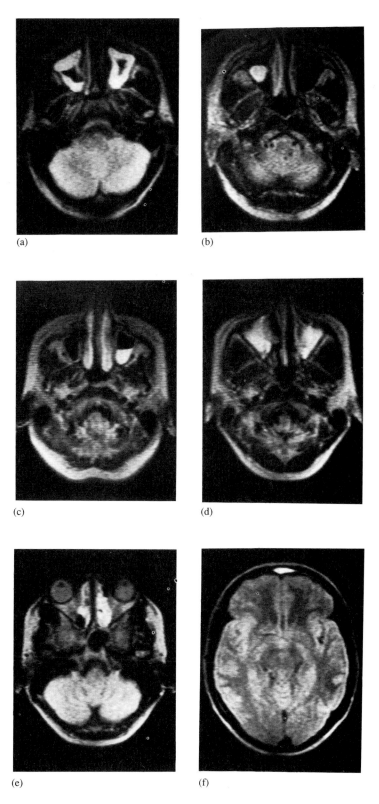

Figure 3.16 Axial MRI scan showing (a) mucosal thickening in both maxillary sinuses; (b) polyp in the right maxillary sinus and enlarged right inferior turbinate; (c) a fluid level in the left maxillary sinus; (d) fluid-filled maxillary, (e) ethmoidal, and (f) frontal sinuses. The fluid in the frontal sinus was confirmed by drainage to be pus. (a), (b) and (c) from Cooke and Hadley (1991)

(a)

(b)

(c)

(d)

(e)

(f)

patients undergoing T_2 weighted axial MRI of the brain had incidental paranasal sinus abnormalities, consider the technique unsuitable for screening individual patients for antral disease. They are of the opinion that it is too expensive and too sensitive, revealing 'normal' changes, such as an asymptomatic retention cyst or thickened sinus mucosa, and should be reserved for specific clinical indications in patients with known or suspected paranasal sinus disease. Cooke and Hadley (1991) examined 483 patients and found evidence of incidental sinus abnormalities in 37.5 per cent but no reliable correlation with symptoms.

Isotope scanning (scintigraphy)

Radioactive isotopes are used diagnostically to demonstrate physiological changes in tissue that often precede anatomical changes, or therapeutically to destroy tumour cells. Bone scans using technetium [$^{99}Tc^m$] phosphate analogues reflect osteoblastic and osteoclastic responses as well as the vascularity of the tissue. The main indication for bone scanning is the search for occult secondary deposits in patients with primary tumours of the lung, breast, prostate, kidney or thyroid, which metastasize to bone.

Extension of an antral carcinoma to involve bone produces an osteoblastic response ahead of the advancing malignant bone destruction. This is evident in the delayed phase of a radionuclide bone scan before bone destruction becomes visible on radiographs. Delayed bone scans have been used to show the generalized bony thickening of Paget's disease, brown tumours of the maxilla secondary to parathyroid carcinoma, a maxillary sinus mucocele extending into the orbit, and ossification of the maxillary sinus 20 years after a Caldwell–Luc operation, and to differentiate localized osteoblastic reaction around an oroantral fistula from osteomyelitis (Noyek, 1979).

Inflammation in bone gives increased tracer uptake but non-purulent inflammation of sinus mucosa does not. If radiographs have shown soft tissue swelling within the sinus, and an isotope scan shows an abnormal focal accumulation of tracer, it indicates either purulent sinusitis or malignancy (Bergstedt and Lind, 1981). Lack of abnormal bony focal accumulation of tracer is indicative of an allergic or vasomotor reaction producing a non-purulent inflammation. Pathological concentration of [$^{99}Tc^m$] diphosphonate may also occur in the maxilla around bone destruction due to chronic periodontitis or periapical disease, and so neither radiology nor scintigraphy is useful for screening for malignant growth in the gingivae (Bergstedt and Lind, 1981).

Ultrasonography

Because the bony facial wall of the sinus is so thin, high power, short duration sound waves from a transmitter are able to pass through it. They are reflected back to the receiver when they hit an impenetrable object.

In sinus sonography a mucosal thickening of the facial wall gives an enlarged first echo peak or a second peak less than 1.5 cm behind the peak from the facial wall. It is diagnostically less accurate than an increased echo from the infratemporal wall, which is an absolute indicator of pathology (Deitmer and Scheffler, 1990). This technique is little used as it gives less information than a sinus radiograph (Pfleiderer, Drake-Lee and Lowe, 1984)

Angiography

Most angiography of the head and neck is via a catheter placed in the femoral artery and guided fluoroscopically into the required vessel.

Sophisticated and precise techniques of cannulation of the external carotid and its maxillary branch can be used to display the arterial supply of facial tumours or vascular anomalies by means of digital subtraction angiography. The abnormal vessels can then be occluded by embolization. Osguthorpe and Hungerford (1983) advocate preoperative embolization of benign osteoblastomas of the maxillary sinus, which are very vascular, to decrease operative blood loss.

Arterial chemotherapy for tumours of the maxillary sinus is no longer practised: a combination of surgery and radiotherapy is preferred.

Biopsy

Any persistent lesion which has no obvious cause should be biopsied. Those contained within the sinus may be sampled via an endoscope. Palatal ulceration may be a late sign of locally invasive antral malignancy and is easily biopsied from an intraoral approach. Ethmoidal polyposis secondary to maxillary sinus neoplasia may resemble benign nasal polyps so all tissue removed from the nose should undergo microscopic examination.

Blood tests

Blood tests give largely non-specific information in sinus disease, though findings such as the grossly raised alkaline phosphatase in Paget's disease or white cell changes in lymphomatous conditions may be diagnostic of particular conditions.

References

Andersen, I., Camner, P., Jensen, P. L., Philipson, K. and Proctor D. F. (1974) Nasal clearance in monozygotic twins. *American Review of Respiratory Disease*, **110**, 301–305

Barrett, C. P., Poliakoff, S. J. and Holder, L. E. (1990) *Primer of Sectional Anatomy with MRI and CT Correlation*, Williams and Wilkins, London

Bergstedt, H. F. and Lind, M. G. (1981) Facial bone scintigraphy VIII. Diagnosis of malignant lesions in the maxillary ethmoidal and palatal bones *Acta Radiologica: Diagnosis*, **22**, 609–618

Bull, T. R. (1987) Examination of the nose: conditions of the external nose. In *Scott-Brown's Otolaryngology*, Vol. 4, 5th edn, (eds I. S. Mackay and T. R. Bull), Butterworth-Heinemann, Oxford, chap. 1

Clement, P. A. R. (1984) Committee report on standardization of rhinomanometry. *Rhinology*, **22**, 151–155

Cooke, L. D. and Hadley, D. M. (1991) MRI of the paranasal sinuses: incidental abnormalities and their relationship to symptoms. *Journal of Laryngology and Otology*, **105**, 278–281

Croft, C. B. (1987) Endoscopy of the nose and sinuses. In *Scott-Brown's Otolaryngology*, Vol. 4, 5th edn (eds I. S. Mackay and T. R. Bull), Butterworth–Heinemann, Oxford, chap. 3

Deitmer, T. and Scheffler, R. (1990) Nasal physiology in swimmers and swimmers' sinusitis. *Acta Otolaryngology*, **110**, 286–291

Ennis, L. M. (1937) Roentgenographic variations of maxillary sinus and nutrient canals of maxilla and mandible. *International Journal of Orthodontia*, **23**, 173–193

Ennis, L. M. and Batson, O. V. (1936) Variations of maxillary sinus as seen in roentgenogram. *Journal of the American Dental Association*, **23**, 201–212

Hallikainen, D. and Paukku, P. (1990) Panoramamic zonography. In *Maxillofacial Imaging* (ed. A Delbalso), W. B. Saunders, Philadelphia, pp. 1–14

Kennedy, D. W., Zinreich, S. J., Rosenbaum, A. E. and Johns, M. E. (1985) Functional endoscopic sinus surgery. Theory and diagnostic evaluation. *Archives of Otolaryngology*, **111**, 576–582

Lauterbur, P. C. (1973) Image formation by induced local interactions: example employing nuclear magnetic resonance. *Nature*, **242**, 190–191

Lund, V. J. (1987) Surgical management of sinusitis. In *Scott-Brown's Otolaringology*, Vol. 4, 5th edn (eds I. S. Mackay and T. R. Bull), Butterworth–Heinemann, Oxford, chap. 11

Mackay, I. and Cole, P. (1987) Rhinitis, sinusitis and associated chest disease. In *Scott-Brown's Otolaringology*, Vol. 4, 5th edn (eds I. S. Mackay and T. R. Bull), Butterworth–Heinemann, Oxford, chap. 6

Marshall, K. G. and Attia, E. L. (1987) *Disorders of the Nose and Paranasal Sinuses. Diagnosis and Management*, PSG, Littleton, MA, pp. 47–53

Moore, J., Potchen, M., Waldenmaier, N., Sierra, A., Potchen, E. J. and Lansing, E. (1986) High-field magnetic resonance imaging of paranasal sinus inflammatory disease. *Laryngoscope*, **96**, 267–271

Moser, F. G., Panush, D., Rubin, J. S., Honigsberg, R. M., Sprayregen, S. and Eisig, S. B. (1991) Incidental paranasal sinus abnormalities on MRI of the brain. *Clinical Radiology*, **43**, 252–254

Newhouse, J. H. and Wiener, J. I. (1991) *Understanding MRI*, Little, Brown, Boston, pp. 35–43

Noyek, A. M. (1979) Bone scanning in otolaryngology. *Laryngoscope*, **89**, (Suppl. 18)

Ohba, T. and Katayama, H. (1976) Comparison of panoramic radiography and Waters' projection in the diagnosis of maxillary sinus disease. *Oral Surgery, Oral Medicine, Oral Pathology*, **42**, 534–588

Osguthorpe, J. D. and Hungerford, G. D. (1983) Benign osteoblastoma of the maxillary sinus. *Head and Neck Surgery*, **6**, 605–609

Paukku, P., Gothlin, J., Totterman, S., Servomaa, A. and Hallikainen, D. (1983a) Radiation doses during panoramic zonography, linear tomography and plain film radiography of maxillofacial skeleton. *European Journal of Radiology*, **3**, 239–241

Paukku, P., Totterman, S., Hallikainen, D., Kinnunen, J. and Gothlin, J. (1983b) Comparison of the visibility of the anatomical structures of the facial skeleton on panoramic zonography and linear tomography. *European Journal of Radiology*, **3**, 177–179

Perez, C. A. and Farman, A. G. (1988) Diagnostic radiology of maxillary sinus defects. *Oral Surgery, Oral Medicine, Oral Pathology*, **66**, 507–512

Pfleiderer, A. G., Drake-Lee, A. B. and Lowe, D. (1984) Ultrasound of the sinuses: a worthwhile procedure? A comparison of ultrasound and radiography in predicting the findings of proof puncture of a maxillary sinus. *Clinical Otolaryngology*, **9**, 335–339

Phelps, P. D. (1987) Radiology of the nose and paranasal sinuses. In *Scott-Brown's Otolaryngology*, Vol. 4, 5th edn (eds I. S. Mackay and T. R. Bull), Butterworth–Heinemann, Oxford, chap. 2

Pogrel, M. A. (1985) Fiberoptic antroscopy. *Journal of Oral and Maxillofacial Surgery*, **43**, 139–142

Rutland, J., Griffin, W. M. and Cole, P. J. (1982) Human ciliary beat frequency in epithelium from intra- and extra-thoracic airways. *American Review of Respiratory Disease*, **125**, 100–105

Smallman, L. A., Hill, S. L. and Stockley R. A. (1984) Reduction of ciliary beat frequencies *in vitro* by sputum from patients with bronchiectasis: a serine proteinase effect. *Thorax*, **39**, 663–667

Southwood, R. (1990) Patient dose reduction in diagnostic radiology. *Report by the Royal College of Radiologists and the National Radiological Protection Board*, **1**, 17

Stammberger, H. and Wolf, G. (1988) Headaches and sinus disease: an endoscopic approach. *Annals of Otology, Rhinology and Laryngology*, **97** (Suppl. 134), 3–23

Sykes, D. A., Wilson, R., Chan, K. L., Mackay, I. S. and Cole, P. J. (1986) Relative importance of antibiotic and improved clearance in topical treatment of chronic mucopurulent rhinosinusits: a controlled study. *Lancet*, **ii**, 359–360

Waters, C. A. and Waldron, M. B. (1915) Roentgenology of the accessory nasal sinuses describing a modification of the occipito-frontal position. *American Journal of Roentgenology*, **2**, 633–639

Westjbal, D. and Kreidler, J. F. (1977) Sinuscopy for the diagnosis of blow out fractures. *Journal of Maxillofacial Surgery*, **5**, 180

White, S. C. and Rose, T. C. (1979) Absorbed bone marrow dose in certain dental radiographic techniques. *Journal of the American Dental Association*, **98**, 553–558

Yanagisawa, E. and Smith, H. W. (1976) Radiology of the normal maxillary sinus and related structures. *Otolaryngologic Clinics of North America*, **9**, 55–81

Chapter 4

Maxillary sinusitis

Maxillary sinusitis is a common disorder and it is therefore useful for dentists to be able to recognize it and provide simple treatment. This chapter will review the problem from a dental perspective; for a more comprehensive medical approach to diseases of the nose and paranasal sinuses readers are recommended to consult an alternative text, such as Marshall and Attia (1987).

The prevalence of maxillary sinusitis is indicated by the fact that it accounts for the loss of half a million working days annually in the UK. The typical triad of sinusitis symptoms is nasal congestion or obstruction, pathological secretion and headache (Messerklinger, 1988). The maxillary teeth and the maxillary sinus lie so close together that it is not surprising that signs and symptoms of disease in one may be confused with signs and symptoms of disease in the other. There are acute and chronic forms, the latter occurring less commonly and often with a history of preceding acute disease. Both conditions affect all age groups, although chronic sinusitis is much less common in children.

Contrary to previous belief, both aerobic and non-aerobic bacteria can be found in apparently healthy sinuses (Brook, 1981) and are similar to those species recovered from infected sinuses. The bacteriology of sinusitis is not as clearly established as might be expected in such a common condition (Arruda *et al.*, 1990; Brook, 1990) because specimens easily become contaminated by nasal organisms. The two species most commonly isolated in acute and chronic sinusitis are *Haemophilus influenzae* and *Streptococcus pneumoniae. H. influenzae* is said to occur more commonly in acute infections and sinusitis in children (Nylen, Jeppson and Branefors-Helander, 1972). However, when suitable techniques are employed, anaerobes are found to predominate in chronic maxillary sinusitis (Su *et al.*, 1983). Unusual organisms occur in unusual circumstances and, for example, *Pseudomonas aeruginosa* is often found in cases with underlying ciliary or mucous disorders, and aspergillosis or mucormycosis in the immune compromised.

Sinusitis of dental origin

Infection of dental origin accounts for a significant proportion of cases of acute sinusitis. The figures in published series vary with the time, the place, the nature of the patient population and the definition of the condition, and range from 5% to 45%. The problem has affected us from prehistoric times (Figure 4.1) but, as dental caries declines and conservative dental care improves, the incidence should reduce.

The dental conditions which may cause maxillary sinusitis are periapical abscess and periapical granuloma, infected dental cysts, oroantral communication, foreign bodies in the antrum and periodontal disease.

Figure 4.1 Abscess on the palatal root of the upper left first molar which has formed a crater-like defect in the sinus floor. Bronze age skull from Orkney, carbon dated at 1100–1300 BC. Specimen by courtesy of Dr Dorothy Lunt, Glasgow Dental School

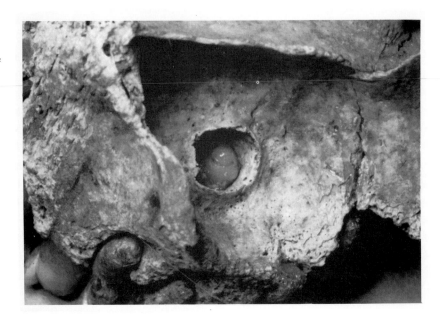

Periapical abscess

The history of acute sinusitis due to discharge of a periapical abscess into the antrum is shorter than that of acute sinusitis of non-odontogenic origin. The symptoms become apparent over a few hours rather than days, and pain from the tooth is likely to precede the onset of the sinusitis. The primary pathogens are anaerobic organisms which originate from the periapical abscess. If the abscess also discharges into the soft tissues of the cheek, it produces a facial swelling, which is unusual in acute sinusitis. Periapical radiographs will confirm the origin (Figures 4.2 and 4.3).

Figure 4.2 Periapical abscess on the palatal root of an upper right first molar which produced an acute purulent maxillary sinusitis

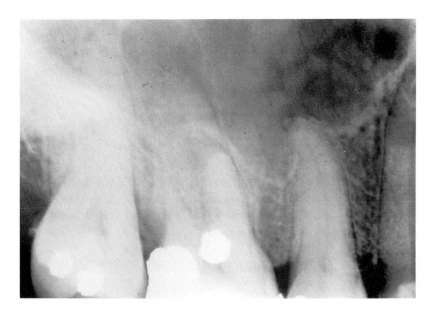

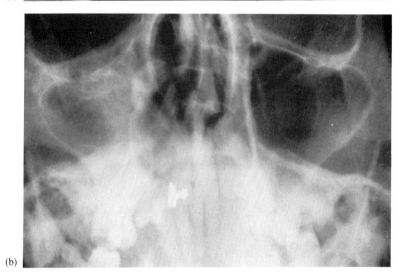

(a)

(b)

Figure 4.3 (a) and (b) Acute maxillary sinusitis from periapical infection of an upper right first molar

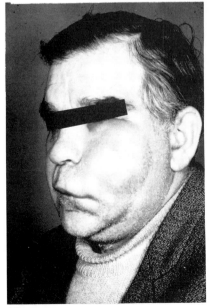

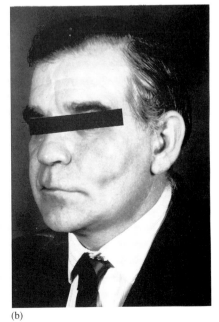

(a)

(b)

Figure 4.4 Severe facial swelling associated with a large infected cyst in the left antrum: (a) the acute phase; (b) the residual swelling after treatment of the acute infection

Treatment in these cases is obviously directed towards the infected tooth. It may be possible to drain the pus through the root canals if the patient is keen to save the tooth but the most reliable method of drainage is extraction. This gives good drainage through a larger opening in the antral floor, and therefore immediate relief of symptoms. Surprisingly, drainage via an extraction socket does not always lead to the formation of a fistula but the possibility must be explained to the patient. Penicillin is effective against most oral anaerobes and is the drug of choice in this situation. Amoxycillin is particularly well absorbed and metronidazole may be used as an adjunct in severe cases. The extraction site should be reviewed and, if a fistula persists, closure should be carried out when the acute sinusitis has resolved (see Chapter 5).

If the acute symptoms have been relieved by drainage through the root canals and antibiotic therapy, the root canals must be prepared and obturated. Care must be taken not to extrude the root filling material into the sinus as this can perpetuate the problem, and has even been associated with antral aspergillosis (Beck-Mannagetta and Necek, 1983).

Infected dental cysts

Cysts which become infected and involve the maxillary sinus can also cause sinusitis (Figure 4.4). They may be apical or dentigerous cysts and are discussed in detail in Chapter 7.

Oroantral fistula

The relationship of oroantral fistulae to chronic sinusitis is explored in Chapter 5.

Dental materials in the antrum

A foreign body is introduced into the sinus during dental treatment when displacement of roots occurs during extraction (see Chapter 5) or if a root canal is overfilled, and sometimes when implants are inserted. Since the materials are inert, an overlong gutta percha point, silver point or a titanium implant does not always cause a reaction in the sinus, and in the absence of symptoms no treatment is necessary. However, if acute or chronic sinusitis develops it will not resolve satisfactorily until the overextended root filling has been removed and the tooth re-treated or extracted (Dodd, Dodds and Holcomb, 1984; Kaplowitz, 1985).

There is a number of published reports of solitary aspergillosis apparently related to excess root filling material in the sinus of otherwise healthy individuals (Beck-Mannagetta and Necek, 1983, 1986; Beck-Mannagetta, Necek and Grasserbauer, 1986). Pastes containing paraformaldehyde and zinc oxide are particularly implicated. The widespread use of such materials, perhaps coupled with a high local prevalence of the infecting fungus, may explain the curiously high numbers of cases reported from Austria (Beck-Mannagetta, Necek and Grasserbauer, 1986).

Implants

Implants are used in the upper edentulous jaw to aid the retention of dentures or bridges, or replace missing teeth. Since one indication for implants is an insufficiency of bone to support a denture, that bone which is present may be very thin and the implants may easily penetrate the nasal or sinus cavities. In a series of clinical cases where implants penetrated the nose or sinus, Brånemark *et al.* (1984) found that the titanium fixtures caused no undesirable side-effects during healing. Implants generally maintained their anchorage during loading but if mobility developed they could be removed and bony healing would take place without fistula formation. The lack of side-effects was attributed to the osseointegration of the implant. Bone and soft tissues have been shown to adhere tightly to the titanium, creating a barrier to micro-organisms or inflammatory processes. The strict sterile technique which is a feature of the Brånemark implant insertion protocol would also reduce the amount of bacterial contamination.

Periodontal disease

Lane and O'Neal (1984) report two cases of chronic sinusitis that resolved following extraction of upper molar teeth which had periodontal disease with trifurcation involvement. In one case the patient had a 5-year history of chronic sinusitis that had failed to respond to antral irrigation and antibiotics. On examination, a communication with the maxillary sinus via a periodontal pocket was demonstrated. After extraction of the involved tooth and periodontal surgery there was no recurrence of sinusitis over a 12-month period.

As the coincident presence of two such common conditions must be frequent, it is difficult to establish an aetiological link. Pressure to extract teeth in sufferers from chronic sinusitis should be resisted, except perhaps in the case of a deep, localized periodontal lesion causing a unilateral sinusitis. However, aggressive periodontal treatment is worth considering when maxillary sinusitis does not resolve after drug therapy. Engstrom *et al.* (1988) demonstrated a convincing relationship between active periodontal disease and antral mucosal thickening observed on periapical radiographs. Thickening was reduced following effective treatment of the periodontal disease. However, radiographic evidence of mucosal thickening (less than 2 mm) is common in asymptomatic individuals (Wilson and Grocutt, 1990).

A case of spontaneous oroantral fistula complicating severe localized periodontitis in a patient positive for the human immunodeficiency virus (HIV) has been reported by Felix *et al.* (1991) (Figure 4.5). The fistula resolved following extraction of two teeth and removal of a sequestrum, though further surgery and antimicrobial therapy was required before the oral ulceration healed.

Acute sinusitis

Non-dental aetiology

Acute maxillary sinusitis involves accumulation of pus in the maxillary sinus and may result from mechanical obstruction of the ostium, direct bacterial contamination, congenitally abnormal clearance mechanisms and immune deficiency, as well as from dental disease (Lund, 1990).

Figure 4.5 Periapical abscess related to the palatal root of the upper left first molar of an HIV positive patient, showing (a) discharge of pus, and (b) partial resolution following sequestration and formation of an oroantral communication. From Felix *et al.* (1991)

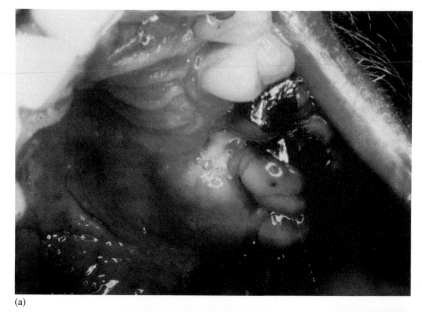

(a)

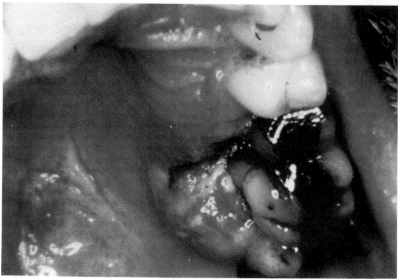

(b)

Mechanical obstruction of the ostium

The most usual cause of ostial obstruction is the common cold. This viral infection produces inflammatory oedema of the nasal mucosa which obstructs the antronasal duct and causes mucus to accumulate in the sinus. Trapped mucus becomes secondarily infected by local commensal bacteria. Direct viral damage to the ciliated cells may also occur and impair drainage.

Allergic rhinitis (hay fever) may cause maxillary discomfort due to oedema round the sinus ostium and retention of secretions, but frank purulent sinusitis is a rare complication (Harland, 1979).

Other conditions which can predispose to mechanical blockage of the ostium, and hence to stagnation and relative anaerobiasis, are deviation of the nasal septum, presence of nasal polyps and prolonged nasotracheal intubation.

Direct bacterial contamination

While this is most frequently from a dental source, infected material may also be introduced directly by jumping or hydrosliding feet first into contaminated water without holding the nose, or during diving, when pressure changes in the nose force nasal secretions into the sinus.

Abnormal clearance mechanisms

Ciliary function is a vital aspect of the normal clearance of maxillary sinus secretions (see Chapter 2). Its failure in primary ciliary dyskinesia (Kartagener's syndrome) or in response to physical or chemical insult will predispose those affected to acute sinusitis. The tenacious mucus in Young's syndrome or in cystic fibrosis sufferers produces the same result. Chronic respiratory tract infection may in itself lead to a vicious circle in which continued microbial burden and the immune response to it damages the cells responsible for mucociliary function (Cole, 1984) (Figure 4.6).

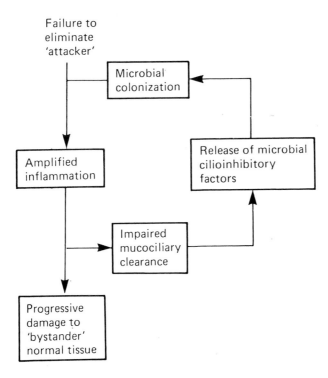

Figure 4.6 Diagram of the vicious circle of chronic inflammation of the respiratory tract. From Mackay and Cole (1987)

Immune deficiency

Sinusitis is known to occur in immune deficiency states, in both congenital abnormalities and acquired conditions, including leukaemias, lymphomas and acquired immunodeficiency syndrome (AIDS), or following the administration of cytotoxic chemotherapy. Sinusitis is not any more prominent than other bacterial infections but may require a more aggressive surgical approach than in normal circumstances. Atypical micro-organisms are commonly found in these cases.

Presenting complaint and history

Typically, there is severe pain located in the cheek and the posterior maxillary teeth, nasal blockage, purulent rhinorrhoea and postnasal drip, with fever and malaise. Pain may be exacerbated by stooping or lowering the head and may be localized to the cheek and maxillary teeth of one side if only one sinus is affected. The pain is often increased by biting on the affected side but is unaffected by drinking hot, cold or sweet fluids. The symptoms are varied and, except when direct bacterial contamination has occurred, arise over a period of days with gradually increasing severity. If the sinusitis arises following a 'cold in the head', symptoms usually start in the recovery period. The dentist should suspect sinusitis as a cause of symptoms if a patient with pain in the upper buccal segments and no obvious dental cause has had a recent upper respiratory tract infection.

There may be a history of a 'cold', but often, even when questioned directly, the patient may not remember any such event. Lack of such a history does not therefore exclude acute sinusitis.

A history of bloody discharge is a potentially sinister sign as it may represent an acute infection of an underlying malignant lesion.

Examination

Extraoral

The general appearance of the face should be assessed, looking particularly for asymmetrical swelling and erythema of the cheeks. There may also be erythema of the skin around the nose and herpes simplex lesions may be present. Inflammatory swelling of the cheeks is extremely rare in acute maxillary sinusitis, unless there is a defect in the anterior sinus wall allowing direct extension of the inflammatory process from the antrum into the cheek.

The cheeks should be palpated bilaterally to detect any tenderness. The maxillary sinus underlies most of the cheek, from below the eye to the roots of the maxillary canine, premolar and molar teeth. As the anterolateral and posterolateral sinus walls are thinnest in the area above the tooth roots, thumb pressure on the cheek here is the best way to elicit tenderness externally. It is perhaps easier to palpate this area intraorally with a finger in the buccal sulcus above the premolars and molars.

A nasal speculum and a headlight are necessary for proper examination of the nasal passages. The nasal mucosa of the anterior nares may show reddening and inflammation and there may even be pus present. Pus from the antronasal duct may be visible under the middle turbinate but it may, of course, have originated from any of the paranasal sinuses of that side.

Intraoral

Careful clinical examination of the teeth, supplemented by thermal or electrical testing and periapical radiography, will identify caries, defective restorations, non-vital or cracked teeth, and acute periapical or periodontal disease. Pain from any of these sources may be confused with sinus pain. Mandibular as well as maxillary teeth should be examined to exclude the possibility of dental pain referred from the lower jaw. Mobility of one or more maxillary molar or premolar teeth, with swelling and tenderness over an apex, usually indicates local dental disease, though it is worth remembering that similar symptoms can be produced by malignant disease within the antrum. Gentle percussion of the maxillary teeth with a mirror handle may elicit tenderness of one or two teeth and suggest a dental source of the problem, but tenderness of a whole buccal segment is indicative of sinusitis.

Pus originating from the maxillary sinus may be seen in the oropharynx as a postnasal drip.

Differential diagnosis

Causes of maxillary pain that are less common than dental or sinus disease include psychogenic facial pain, trigeminal or other neuralgias, and temporo-mandibular joint disorders.

Radiology and other investigations

Radiographs of the maxillary sinuses taken early in an acute episode of sinusitis may show no abnormality. This is because sufficient swelling of the lining and retention of secretions to produce radiographic changes take a few days to develop. Radiographs may be unnecessary if the diagnosis is obvious on clinical grounds and the sinusitis resolves after appropriate treatment. However, an acute episode of sinusitis occasionally masks an underlying carcinoma, especially in an older patient. Some patients who become symptom free have residual pus in the antrum; this can be identified radiographically and drained to advantage.

The occipitomental view (Waters' projection), taken in the upright position, is usually the radiograph of choice. This view shows both maxillary sinuses and therefore allows comparison of the two sides and correlation with the symptoms (Figure 4.3b). Bleeding into the sinus following facial trauma produces the same appearance so this possibility needs to be borne in mind. CT scanning demonstrates mucosal abnormalities in the nose and sinuses very clearly (Figure 4.7). Periapical, occlusal or panoramic views may be of use in identifying a dental cause for the acute sinusitis (Figure 4.2, 4.3a). Advanced periodontal disease, recurrent caries leading to pulp death and apical abscess, extruded root filling material or ruptured apical cysts can all produce acute sinusitis and are best identified using periapical radiographs to supplement clinical examination.

Figure 4.7 Widespread gross mucosal thickening of the nasal and sinus mucosa demonstrated by CT scanning

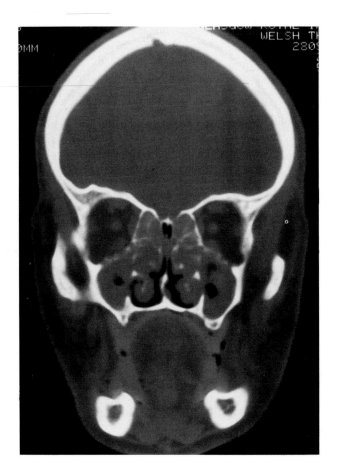

If radiological appearances are equivocal, proof puncture via the interior meatus, or the canine fossa, is useful for providing material for bacteriological culture and sensitivity. While *S. pneumoniae* and *H. influenzae* are commonly recovered from cases of acute sinusitis, it is probable that, as in the case of dentoalveolar abscess, this mainly reflects contamination due to the isolation methods in use, and other significant pathogens, particularly strict anaerobes, are under-recognized.

Direct visualization of the sinus mucosa by antroscopy through the canine fossa will absolutely confirm the diagnosis and this is a technique which could be used to advantage more commonly. As well as visualization of the mucosa it provides the opportunity for more meaningful bacteriological investigation.

Treatment of acute sinusitis

The keystones of therapy are the provision of drainage to remove the pus and to re-aerate the sinus mucosa, and removal of the cause. Failure to do either effectively can lead to establishment of a chronic sinusitis.

Drainage is preferably achieved by supporting and restoring the natural drainage mechanism through the antronasal duct with antibiotics and nasal decongestants. However, if the cause is dental, drainage is achieved at the same time as the cause is removed by root canal therapy or extraction of the offending tooth. The communication may heal spontaneously and an oroantral fistula does not inevitably follow extraction in this situation.

The physiological drainage mechanisms, described in Chapter 2, are disrupted in acute sinusitis because ciliary activity is reduced or disorientated by bacterial toxins, the mucous blanket is diluted or swamped by serous secretions, and swelling of the mucosa lining the ostium or antronasal duct may partially or completely block the passage of secretions into the nose. This last factor provides the rationale for the use of decongestant nasal drops containing sympathomimetic drugs. The vasoconstriction of the nasal mucosa and antral fontanelles reduces vascular engorgement and therefore reduces the mucosal swelling. Patients have to be shown how to hold the head in a dependent position (Figure 4.8), before instilling the drops, to prevent the fluid running straight into the pharynx.

Ephedrine nasal drops (0.5%) are most commonly used and can give relief for several hours. One or two drops instilled 8-hourly are usually adequate. There is danger of an interaction with the now infrequently used monoamine oxidase inhibitor antidepressants, precipitating a hypertensive crisis, so this concurrence should be avoided. Rebound secondary vasodilatation can occur following the

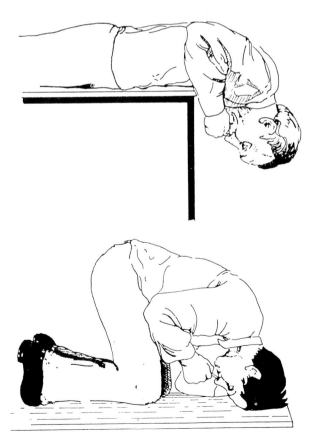

Figure 4.8 The head down and forwards position for instilling nasal drop medication. From Mackay and Cole (1987)

use of nasal decongestants. The consequent temporary increase in nasal congestion encourages the patient to use further decongestant, thus establishing a vicious circle of events. Use for longer than 10–14 days produces persistent mucosal oedema and severe nasal obstruction (rhinitis medicamentosa). Xylometazoline (0.1%) is an alternative to ephedrine but is perhaps more likely to cause a rebound effect. Systemic nasal decongestants are of no proved value.

Effective antibiotics include doxycycline hydrochloride (Vibramycin) 100 mg daily, following a loading dose of 200 mg, for adults. Penicillin, amoxycillin or co-trimoxazole may also be used and are preferred for children, to avoid discoloration of the developing teeth. Antibacterial chemotherapy alone is insufficient treatment of sinusitis.

Steam inhalations may act by hydrating the mucous blanket, making it less viscous and thereby encouraging normal ciliary clearance of the maxillary sinus. The use of volatile aromatic additives, such as menthol or eucalyptus, may encourage patients' compliance since they stimulate cold-receptor nerve endings, producing the illusion of coolness and therefore an illusion of improvement in nasal air flow. A suitable steam inhalation is Menthol and Eucalyptus Inhalation BP, one teaspoonful of which is added to a pint of hot (not boiling) water in a bowl, and the vapour inhaled using a towel to form a 'tent' over the head and bowl. It is advisable to use an old container for dissolving the crystals as the solution produces a stain which is not easily removed! Steam inhalations are a traditional and comforting adjunct with at least a placebo effect.

If antibiotics and nasal drops fail to resolve the condition, pus must be removed from the antrum in order to allow the sinus mucosa to recover and the self-cleansing mechanisms to be re-established.

Pus is removed by antral lavage, which may need to be repeated several times on a weekly basis until clear fluid rather than mucopus is returned in the washings. In adults the procedure is carried out under local anaesthesia by inserting a hollow trochar and cannula into the antrum through the nasal wall beneath the inferior turbinate (see Figure 3.1). Warmed normal saline is syringed through the cannula and the fluid and pus return via the antronasal duct. Antibiotics and nasal decongestants are subsequently prescribed and this should produce resolution of disease and return of normal function.

Further surgical management of recurrent acute sinusitis includes inferior meatal antrostomy, and formerly middle meatal antrostomy, but if the cause of infection has not been eliminated the antral lining cannot recover and symptoms will persist. The most common complication is the development of chronic sinusitis. This arises due to failure to remove a source of infection, a foreign body or any accumulated pus promptly, following irreversible damage to the antral lining or in the presence of an underlying systemic condition.

Complications

Serious complications from spreading infection from acute maxillary sinusitis are now rare because most severe infections are treated promptly and effectively. The direction of spread which is most dangerous is to the orbit, often by way of an associated ethmoidal sinusitis – which indeed may have preceded the maxillary infection. Orbital swelling, pain and loss of vision are signs which should prompt ophthamological investigation (Watson, Dick and Hutchinson, 1991) and urgent treatment, including large dose intravenous antibiotic therapy and surgical drainage (Robbins and Tarshis, 1981).

Chronic sinusitis

Definition and diagnosis

The term 'chronic sinusitis' is poorly defined but is best considered as persistent, incompletely resolved acute sinusitis. A distinction is sometimes made between the recurrent acute and the chronic forms, implying that surgery is indicated in the latter case to deal with irreversible changes in the antral mucosa which are unresponsive to conservative treatment (Marshall and Attia, 1987). However, it is also commonly due to the persistence of external aggravating factors such as nasal polyposis, septal deviation and allergic rhinitis, which impair ventilation and drainage, and even perhaps chronic marginal periodontitis, which can cause antral mucosal thickening (Engstrom *et al.*, 1988).

Melen *et al.* (1986) suggest that the diagnosis should be based on duration of symptoms, the results of ear, nose and throat and dental examinations, sinus radiographs and/or sinoscopy and conservative treatment. Symptoms should have persisted or have reappeared over a period of 3 months, and sinus radiographs or sinoscopy demonstrated persistent local or generalized mucosal swelling. Chronic nasal obstruction, a long-standing purulent nasal discharge, headache, facial pain or a sensation of pressure and a dull ache over the sinuses, together with history of previous sinusitis, all suggest chronic sinusitis.

Chronic maxillary sinusitis of dental origin has been associated with oroantral fistula, non-vital teeth, inflammatory periapical or periodontal lesions, and even the follicles of impacted teeth involved in a periodontal or periapical lesion. A dental cause accounted for 40% of the cases of chronic maxillary sinusitis studied by Melen *et al.* (1986).

Proof puncture and subsequent culture may reveal a causative organism resistant to antibiotic therapy previously prescribed. Bacteriological cultures of samples of antral mucosa recovered at operation (Su *et al.*, 1983) suggest that anaerobes are the most important pathogens in chronic maxillary sinusitis because they were only isolated in inflamed mucosa, whereas aerobes were found in the absence of inflammation.

Treatment of chronic sinusitis

Sound treatment must depend on identification of the cause of the chronic sinusitis. Removal of local factors such as a dental cause, the cause of ostium obstruction or the source of direct bacterial contamination, together with control of any infection present, should effect a cure. However, underlying systemic conditions compromising mucociliary clearance mechanisms or immune competence may make effective treatment difficult.

Antrostomy

Inferior meatal antrostomy was used in the treatment of chronic sinusitis by 78% of British otolaryngologists surveyed by Lund (1986). With this method it is hoped the damaged mucosa will return to normal by a combination of aeration and gravitational drainage.

In the past, and particularly before the advent of antibiotics, removal of the 'irreversibly' damaged antral lining, and creation of a nasal antrostomy under general anaesthesia, was commonly achieved by a Caldwell–Luc operation. The procedure was described independently by Caldwell (1893), Spicer (1894) and Luc (1897) and its popularity has waxed and waned since then as surgical fashion has favoured alternately the nasal and the buccal approach to antrostomy. The unhealthy lining is completely stripped from the antral walls, and the objective is healing with healthy fibrous tissue. An antrostomy is created into the inferior meatus, to allow immediate postoperative drainage and aeration of the sinus, and the intraoral incision is closed. Supportive treatment with antibiotics, nasal drops and steam inhalations is prescribed.

A straight incision is made in the reflection of the buccal sulcus from the lateral incisor to the first molar and can be extended further if required. An incision along the gingival margin of the upper teeth may also be used, or, in the edentulous patient, an incision slightly buccal to the crest of the ridge with a relieving incision anteriorly into the labial sulcus. The incision is placed slightly buccally to an edentulous ridge to avoid discomfort from a scar directly beneath the area taking the maximum denture load. The mucoperiosteum is reflected apically, care being taken to avoid stretching the infraorbital nerve, and a window of bone distal to the canine root, in the canine fossa, is outlined and removed. Instead of removing this bone, Sanderson (1983) suggests that it is preferable to try to create the opening using an osteoplastic flap hinged above on the antral mucosa.

The radical removal of antral mucosa is no longer favoured as a routine, and the antrostomy is also criticized because it, too, interferes with the normal mechanisms of sinus drainage. The removal of bone from the facial wall of the sinus to provide access produces a defect, covered only with scar tissue. The larger this defect is made in the interest of good access, the more the volume of the maxillary sinus will be reduced postoperatively by the inward collapse of the soft tissue of the cheek. Contraction of tissue near the site of the infraorbital nerve may also lead to neurogenic pain. However, the requirements for generous surgical access to the maxillary sinus necessary, for example, for removal of a displaced tooth (see Chapter 5) outweigh these disadvantages, and the complications are relatively minor in most cases.

Transnasal endoscopic surgery

The development of fibreoptic technology and endoscopy has made an alternative approach to sinus surgery possible. Messerklinger (1978) and Stammberger (1989) advocate an endoscopic approach to the middle meatus using a rigid instrument to visualize the infundibulum and the natural openings of the sinuses. This can reveal the presence of bony distortions, nasal mucosal thickening or polyps, and also the source of discharge of pus. Based on precise diagnosis, corrective surgery and access for drainage of the ethmoid sinuses can be achieved. These techniques, while exacting in the requirement for special equipment and training, are associated with less morbidity than traditional methods. Access to the maxillary sinus is easily gained from the buccal approach but the reservoir of persistent infection may lie in the other, more inaccessible sinuses.

Maxillary sinusitis in children

The developing maxillary sinuses are smaller than those of the adult and have a less unfavourable gravitational drainage site (see Chapter 1). The deciduous teeth are separated from the sinus by the permanent tooth germs and are therefore less likely to cause infection.

Both acute and chronic maxillary sinusitis are less common in children than in adults, but they do occur and with potentially very serious consequences. Brook *et al.* (1980) reported two cases, one in a six-year-old boy and the other in a nine-year-old girl, where periapical abscesses of the previously traumatized upper incisors spread to involve the maxillary and ethmoid sinuses. Both patients had periorbital cellulitis and culture revealed the presence of anaerobic organisms. Treatment involved surgical drainage of both the maxillary sinus and the alveolar abscess, and the administration of intravenous and then oral antibiotics.

Fungal Infections

Aspergillosis

Aspergillus is an airborne spore-forming fungus found in soil and decaying vegetable matter, and in certain circumstances it may become pathogenic in man. The most frequent infecting species is *A. fumigatus* and both localized and invasive infections are described. Healthy individuals have a solitary localized lesion (Meikle, Yarington and Winterbauer, 1985) but patients with debilitating illness are susceptible to a potentially lethal infection, characterized by generalized progressive tissue destruction (Shannon, Schlaroff and Colm, 1990). Clinically and radiologically the non-destructive form is indistinguishable from non-specific chronic sinusitis, but the destructive form mimics neoplastic disease and presents similar management problems (De Foer, Fossion and Vaillant, 1990). Coexistence of aspergillosis and squamous cell carcinoma in the maxillary sinus was reported by Tanaka *et al.* (1985), who speculated on the possibility of malignant change arising in squamous cell metaplasia produced by aspergillosis, while being unable to rule out secondary infection of a spontaneously arising carcinoma. Treatment of the solitary aspergillosis consists of removal of the mycotic mass. As the antral mucosa remains largely intact, antimycotic therapy is considered unnecessary.

Beck-Mannagetta and Necek (1986) showed by chemical analysis that radiopaque masses observed in patients with solitary aspergillosis of the maxillary sinus consisted of zinc oxide cement from overfilled teeth. In a series of 30 otherwise healthy patients, aged 19–63 years, who developed aspergillosis, one had a chronic oroantral fistula and all the rest had received endodontic therapy. Zinc alone, or contained in zinc oxide, and other metal ions stimulated growth of *A. fumigatus in vitro.*

In order to prevent antral aspergillosis, any excess zinc oxide containing root filling materials should be carefully removed. In the absence of endodontic material, the mycotic infection could still be explained by a previously extracted endodontically treated tooth, the former presence of root filling material in the antrum which has been expelled via the ostium, or simply by chronic inhalation of spore-bearing dust.

Mucormycosis

Mucormycosis or phycomycosis is a rare fungal infection but it is reported with increasing frequency in immunocompromised patients and is potentially lethal (Esakowitz *et al.*, 1987; Toriumi, Rosenfeld and Pelzer, 1988). It occurs in two main forms: superficial and visceral.

The visceral form, which affects the head and neck, is of most interest to dental surgeons and will be discussed here. It is commonly accompanied by a triad of symptoms: uncontrolled diabetes mellitus, periorbital infection and meningoencephalitis. The most common predisposing factor is poorly controlled diabetes mellitus, although cases have been reported in association with malignant lymphomas, and after administration of steroids, antimetabolites and antibiotics.

The disease is probably transmitted by inhalation and extends from the nasal cavity into the paranasal sinuses, orbit and cranial cavity by direct invasion of vascular channels (Breiman, Sadowsky and Friedman, 1981). Thrombosis and haemorrhagic ischaemia occur, producing a marked inflammatory response in the involved tissues.

Signs and symptoms of the disease are similar to those of sinus carcinoma and may be indistinguishable clinically and radiologically. There may be dark, bloody nasal discharge and necrosis of the nasal turbinates, ptosis and proptosis, ophthalmoplegia, loss of vision, trigeminal anaesthesia and facial palsy.

Treatment of mucormycosis involves control of the underlying predisposing factor, surgical excision if the lesion is localized, and antibiotic therapy, the drug of choice being amphotericin B. Even so, the disease can spread rapidly and result in a fatal mycotic infection.

References

Arruda, L. K., Sole, D., Weckx, L. L. M., Naspitz, C. K. and Mimica, I. M. (1990) Bacterial flora of 'normal' sinuses. *Pediatrics*, **86**, 649

Beck-Mannagetta, J. and Necek, D. (1983) Solitary aspergillosis of maxillary sinus, a complication of dental treatment. *Lancet*, **ii**, 1260

Beck-Mannagetta, J. and Necek, D. (1986) Radiologic findings in aspergillosis of the maxillary sinus. *Oral Surgery, Oral Medicine, Oral Pathology*, **62**, 345–349

Beck-Mannagetta, J., Necek, D. and Grasserbauer, M. (1986) Zahnärztliche Aspekte der Solitären Kieferhöhlen–Aspergillose. *Zeitschrift für Stomatologie*, **83**, 283–315

Brånemark, P. I., Adell, R., Albrektsson, T., Lekholm, U., Lindstrom, J. and Rockler, B. (1984) An experimental and clinical study of osseointegrated implants penetrating the nasal cavity and maxillary sinus. *Journal of Oral and Maxillofacial Surgery*, **42**, 497–505

Breiman, A., Sadowsky, D. and Friedman, J. (1981) Mucormycosis. Discussion and report of a case involving the maxillary sinus. *Oral Surgery, Oral Medicine, Oral Pathology*, **52**, 375–378

Brook, I. (1981) Aerobic and anaerobic bacterial flora of normal maxillary sinuses. *Laryngoscope*, **91**, 372–376

Brook, I. (1990) Bacterial flora of 'normal' sinuses. *Pediatrics*, **86**, 649

Brook, I., Friedman, E. M., Rodriguez, W. J. and Controni, G. (1980) Complications of sinusitis in children. *Pediatrics*, **66**, 568–572

Caldwell, G. W. (1893) Diseases of the accessory sinuses of the nose and an infrared method of treatment of suppuration of the maxillary antrum. *New York Medical Journal*, **58**, 526–528

Cole, P. J. (1984) A new look at the pathogenesis and management of persistent bronchial sepsis. In *Strategies for the Management of Chronic Bronchial Sepsis* (ed. R. J. Davies), Medicine Publishing Foundation, Oxford, pp.1–20

De Foer, C., Fossion, E. and Vaillant, J. M. (1990) Sinus aspergillosis. *Journal of Cranio-Maxillo-Facial Surgery*, **18**, 33–40

Dodd, R. B., Dodds, R. N. and Holcomb, J. B. (1984) An endodontically induced maxillary sinusitis. *Journal of Endodontics*, **10**, 504–506

Engstrom, H., Chamberlain, D., Kiger, R. and Egelberg, J. (1988) Radiographic evaluation of the effect of initial periodontal therapy on thickness of the maxillary sinus mucosa. *Journal of Periodontology*, **59**, 604–608

Esakowitz, L., Cook, S. D., Adams, J. *et al.* (1987) Rhino-orbital-cerebral mucormycosis – a clinico-pathological report of two cases. *Scottish Medical Journal*, **32**, 180–182

Felix, D. H., Wray, D., Smith, G. L. F. and Jones, G. A. (1991) Oro-antral fistula: an unusual complication of HIV-associated periodontal disease. *British Dental Journal*, **171**, 61–62

Harland, R. W. (1979) The management of hayfever in general practice. *Journal of the Royal College of General Practitioners*, **29**, 265–286

Kaplowitz, (1985) Penetration of the maxillary sinus by overextended gutta percha cones. Report of two cases. *Clinical Preventive Dentistry*, **7(2)**, 28–30

Lane, J. J. and O'Neal, R. B. (1984) The relationship between periodontitis and the maxillary sinus. *Journal of Periodontology*, **55**, 477–481

Luc, H. (1897) Une nouvelle méthode opératoire pour la cure radicale et rapide de l'empyeme chirurgique de sinus maxillaire. *Archives Internationales de Laryngologie, d'Otologie et de Rhinologie*, **10**, 273–285

Lund, V. J. (1986) The design and function of intranasal antrostomies. *Journal of Laryngology and Otology*, **100**, 35–39

Lund, V. J. (1990) Sinusitis. *Prescribers' Journal*, **30**, 212–217

Mackay, I. and Cole, P. (1987) Rhinitis, sinusitis and associated chest disease. In *Scott-Brown's Otolaryngology*, Vol. 4, 5th edn (eds I. S. Mackay and T. R. Bull), Butterworth–Heinemann, Oxford, chap. 6

Marshall, K. G. and Attia, E. L. (1987) *Disorders of the Nose and Paranasal Sinuses. Diagnosis and Management*. PSG, Littleton, MA

Meikle, D., Yarington, C. T. and Winterbauer, R. M. (1985) Aspergillosis of the maxillary sinuses in otherwise healthy patients. *Laryngoscope*, **95**, 776–779

Melen, I., Lindahl, L., Andreasson, L. and Rundcrantz, H. (1986) Chronic maxillary sinusitis. Definition, diagnosis and relation to dental infection and nasal polyposis. *Acta Otolaryngologica (Stockholm)*, **101**, 320–327

Messerklinger (1978) *Endoscopy of the nose*. Urban and Schwertzenberg, Baltimore/Munich

Nylen, O., Jeppson, P. H. and Branefors-Helander, P. (1972) Acute sinusitis. *Scandinavian Journal of Infectious Disease*, **4**, 43–48

Robbins, K. T., and Tarshis, L. M. (1981) Blindness: a complication of odontogenic sinusitis. *Otolaryngology and Head and Neck Surgery*, **89**, 938–940

Sanderson, B. A. (1983) Physiologic maxillary antrostomy – an update. *Laryngoscope*, **93**, 180–183

Shannon, M. T., Schlaroff, A. and Colm, S. J. (1990) Invasive aspergillosis of the maxilla in an immunocomprised patient. *Oral Surgery, Oral Medicine, Oral Pathology*, **70**, 425–427

Spicer, S. (1894) The surgical treatment of chronic emphyema of the antrum maxillaire. *BMJ*, **2**, 1359

Su, W. -Y., Liu, C., Hung, S. -Y. and Tsai, W. -F. (1983) Bacteriological study in chronic maxillary sinusitis. *Laryngoscope*, **93**, 931–934

Stammberger (1989) *Functional Endoscopic Nasal and Perinasal Sinus Surgery – The Messerklinger Technique*. B. C. Deeker, Toronto/Philadelphia

Tanaka, T., Nishioka, K., Naito, M., Masuda, Y. and Ogura, Y. (1985) Co-existence of aspergillosis and squamous cell carcinoma in the maxillary sinus proven by preoperative cytology. *Acta Cytologica*, **29,** 73–78

Toriumi, D. M., Rosenfeld, S. and Pelzer, H. J. Jr (1988) Residents' page. Pathologic quiz case 1. *Archives of Otolaryngology and Head and Neck Surgery*, **114,** 1190–1192

Watson, N. J., Dick, A. D. and Hutchinson, C. H. (1991) A case of sinusitis presenting with sphenocavernous syndrome: discussion of the differential diagnosis. *Scottish Medical Journal*, **36,** 179–180

Wilson, P. S. and Grocutt, M. (1990) Mucosal thickening on sinus X-ray and its significance. *Journal of Laryngology and Otology*, **104,** 694–695

Chapter 5

Traumatic penetration

The anatomy of the maxillary sinus and its relationship to the surrounding structures has been detailed in Chapter 1. As a result of this relationship, the sinus may be directly involved in tooth extraction, leading to an oroantral communication, sometimes further complicated by displacement of a root. Fracture of the maxillary tuberosity may also occur and produce a large opening into the sinus. Zygomatic complex, orbital floor and middle-third fractures inevitably involve it, and it is exposed during maxillary down-fracture procedures for correction of facial deformities.

Oroantral fistula

Definition

A fistula is defined as an abnormal communication between two internal organs, or between an internal organ and the surface of the body. An oroantral fistula is therefore an abnormal communication between the oral cavity and the maxillary sinus.

Incidence

Ehrl (1980) reviewed all extractions and closures of oroantral communications over a 9-year period in Hessen, Germany, and found that 1 in 180 first molar extractions and 1 in 280 second molar extractions resulted in perforation of the antrum. These figures related only to those cases in which communication was recognized, so the true frequency is probably higher.

Aetiology and prevention

Oroantral communication is more likely to occur when there is periapical pathology, a large antrum or a lone-standing molar; in younger patients, where the antrum is not fully formed, it is most unlikely.

Thick buccal bone overlying an upper first molar in an intact arch may come away with the tooth, resulting in a communication. The authors have seen a considerable defect produced when premolars and molars together with the surrounding bone were removed *en bloc* during an excessively forceful extraction. If unusual resistance is encountered during extraction it is better to resort to surgical bone removal or division of the tooth than to apply further force.

Elderly patients with few remaining maxillary teeth may appear to have larger sinuses than younger persons. This is partly due to increased pneumatization of the sinuses but is mainly a result of the considerable alveolar resorption associated with loss of teeth. Extraction in these cases should be undertaken with extra care and the patient must be warned that it may be impossible to avoid communication with the antrum (Figure 5.1). Preoperative radiographic examination may prompt a warning to the patient and perhaps encourage extra care, but otherwise does not alter the risk of perforating the antrum (Figure 5.2).

Pathogenesis

Some communications will close spontaneously, but prediction is difficult. In a study of 104 perforations of the maxillary sinus, von Wowern (1970) concluded that the chance of spontaneous healing was small and that therefore closure of a sinus perforation is always indicated. Closure within the first 48 hours reduces the chances of infection and the development of chronic changes in the antral mucosa and is associated with faster healing and a higher success rate.

Diagnosis

All extracted upper posterior teeth should be examined, not only to ensure that they are intact but also for indications of a sinus communication. If the roots are covered with a thin plate of bone, or adherent sinus mucosa, a communication must be present.

The patient should be asked to attempt to blow air into the pinched nose with the mouth open. This forces air into the maxillary sinus via its ostium. If an oroantral defect is present, bubbles appear in the extraction socket. A false negative result may be obtained if thickened antral lining or polyps temporarily occlude the communication, or indeed the ostium. Gentle probing of the socket with a blunt instrument, such as a ball-ended periodontal probe or small amalgam plugger, will confirm the bone defect without perforating an intact lining.

Figure 5.1 Oroantral communication was correctly predicted from this pre-extraction radiograph but was closed successfully by advancing a buccal flap

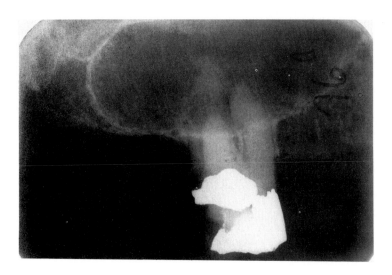

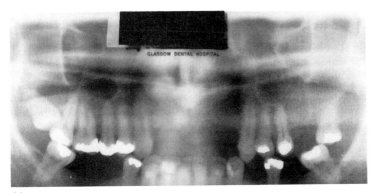

(a)

Figure 5.2 (a) Removal of the upper right third molar led to (b) an oroantral fistula and (c) the area of chronic sinusitis. Because of the close proximity of the second molar two operations were required before closure was achieved.

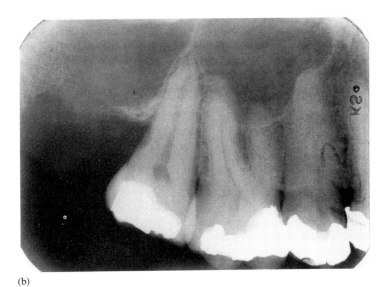

(b)

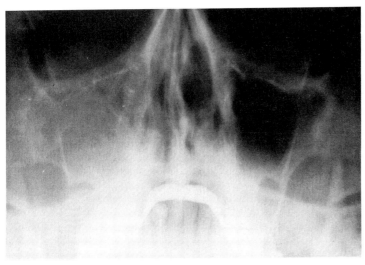

(c)

Figure 5.3 Oroantral fistula produced by extraction of the upper right first molar. The socket outline is seen to communicate with the deficit in the sinus floor

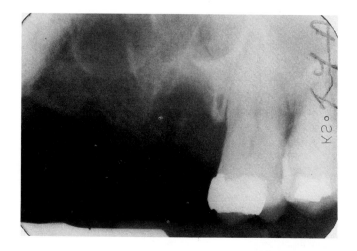

Figure 5.4 Chronic oroantral fistula of 22 years' standing. Symptoms were only mild and intermittent. The mucosal thickening is no worse in the left than in the uninvolved right sinus

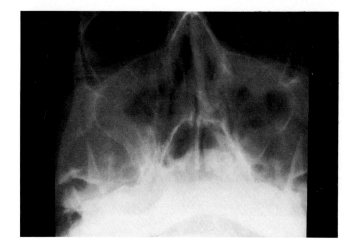

Figure 5.5 Bilateral oroantral fistulae of 1 year's standing. The patient at first refused operation for fear of general anaesthesia. When eventually persuaded to have surgical closure the left sinus, which had the larger opening, contained a number of green peas!

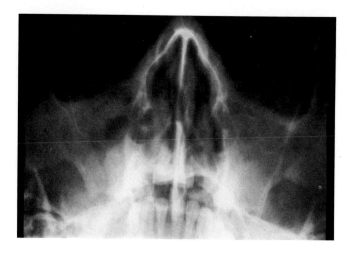

Radiography

Radiographs are unnecessary following oroantral fistula formation, provided the entire tooth has been removed, but are useful to determine whether a dislodged root is in the antrum, in the socket, or beneath the buccal or palatal mucosa, and also to record the radiographic appearance of the sinus at the time (Figure 5.3).

Chronic oroantral fistula

An unrecognized or unsuccessfully treated communication can become a chronic fistula. When present for over a month, the tract will be completely epithelialized and there can be no expectation of spontaneous closure.

The patient may complain of a foul taste or smell, passage of food or drink into the nose, symptoms of chronic sinusitis, inability to 'draw' on a cigarette or pipe, or blow a wind instrument, or may be asymptomatic.

Larger defects may be less troublesome and asymptomatic because the opening into the mouth allows drainage of the sinus, whereas smaller defects are more likely to become blocked and produce symptoms of sinusitis (Figure 5.4 and 5.5).

A small dimple on the alveolar ridge may be the only sign (Figure 5.6), or there may be an obvious defect or an associated lump of granulation tissue, prolapsed lining or polyp protruding from the fistula (Figure 5.7). Pus may be visible at the mouth of the opening or be released on probing the socket. The diagnostic steps outlined above should be followed.

Biopsy is indicated if there is any suspicion of malignancy as antral carcinoma may present in this way (Figure 5.8).

Drainage and irrigation will facilitate resolution of any sinusitis. To promote drainage, the oroantral fistula can be enlarged by excising a margin of surrounding mucosa, by cauterizing any granulation tissue and polyps protruding from the sinus with electrocoagulation, or simply by cautious application of a chemical agent such as trichloracetic acid. The patient is provided with a syringe and blunted wide-bore needle, or a plastic irrigating tube, to wash out the sinus with warm salt water three or four times daily, and a course of amoxycillin is prescribed. Once the antral washings are clear and the symptoms have subsided, closure can be carried out as described below.

The antral mucosa usually recovers after the elimination of the fistula, so radical removal of the sinus mucosa and nasal antrostomy are rarely, if ever, required (Lund, 1986).

Treatment

The aim of treatment of a communication created by extraction is to provide support for the socket blood clot so it will organize, be replaced by bone, and epithelialize on its oral and antral surfaces.

Provided there is no purulent discharge, the oroantral communication should be closed as soon as it is recognized. No material should be put into the socket as this will delay healing.

If the patient is to be referred for treatment, the clot in the defect may be protected with a dressing of ribbon gauze soaked in Whitehead's varnish

Figure 5.6 Chronic oroantral fistula (a) mucosal defect demonstrated by a probe and (b) the underlying bony defect revealed at surgery which, as always, is much larger. A silver point root filling can be seen protruding from the premolar apex

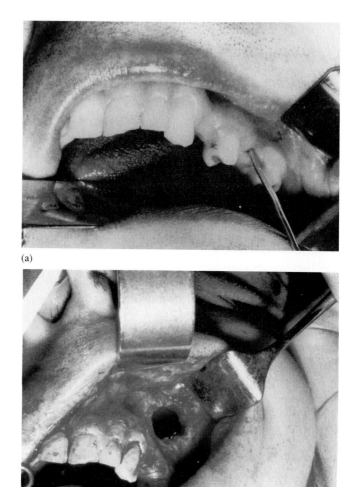

(a)

(b)

Figure 5.7 Antral lining prolapsed through a large chronic fistula in the second molar area

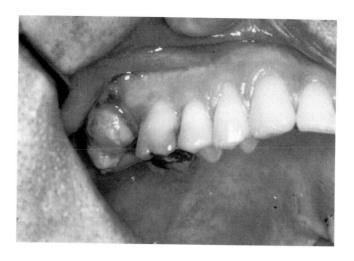

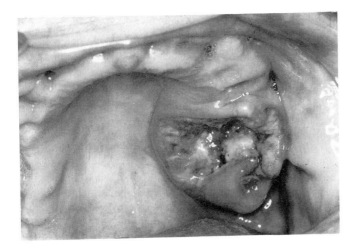

Figure 5.8 Exuberant tissue growth in an upper molar socket some weeks after an upper clearance. Clinical suspicion of malignancy was confirmed by biopsy

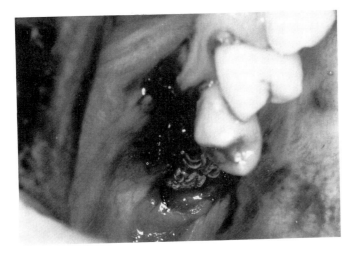

Figure 5.9 Patient referred for advice after creation of an oroantral communication during the extraction of two upper molars. The defect has been covered by suturing the buccal and palatal socket margins together and placing a ribbon gauze patch. Despite the rather untidy repair the outcome was extremely satisfactory and sound closure was achieved

(Iodoform paint, BP) sutured over it (Figure 5.9), or with an acrylic splint. If making a splint, a piece of gauze or metal foil should be placed over the socket to prevent impression material being forced into the antrum. Complete closure of a communication created within the previous 48 hours can be obtained in this way. The splint is a useful additional support for the healing tissues in patients who are heavy smokers. The negative intraoral pressure created when drawing on a cigarette seems to aggravate wound breakdown, and there may even be a direct effect from the tobacco smoke.

When there has been loss of alveolar bone without loss of soft tissue, closure may be achievable by suturing the buccal and palatal gingival margins together. Usually, however, there is insufficient readily available mucosa and a different method of closure has to be used to support the blood clot while healing takes place. The most successful methods are the buccal advancement flap and the palatal rotation flap. Other methods have been described, including the use of implantable material, to cover the defect. The advantage is that less extensive surgery is required and this may be easier for the inexperienced. However, except for the collagen implant (Mitchell and Lamb, 1983), a second operation is required to remove the material. Any flap used to cover a bony defect should have a good blood supply and the suture line should lie on undamaged bone. When a tooth adjacent to a fistula has an exposed root and has lost its supporting bone, there may be difficulty in obtaining a satisfactory closure and the tooth may have to be sacrificed.

The buccal advancement flap, first described by Rehrmann (1936), is most commonly used because of its reliability and the relatively easy surgical technique (Figure 5.10). The palatal flap is used much less frequently. Very

Figure 5.10 (a)–(d) The buccal advancement flap technique.

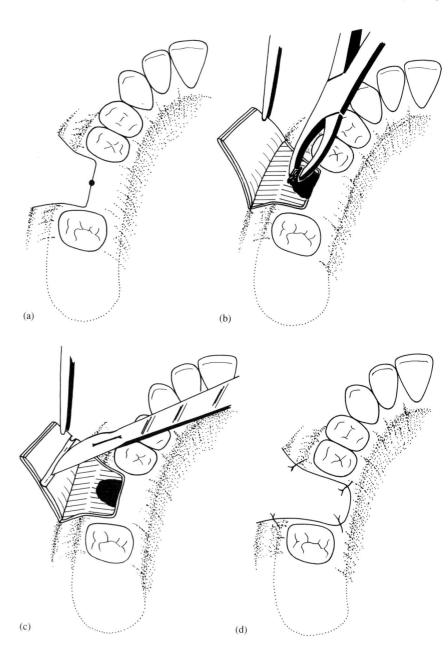

(a)

(b)

(c)

(d)

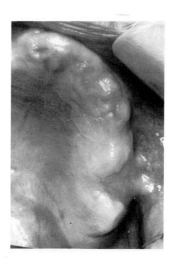

Figure 5.11 The sulcus defect produced by advancement of a buccal flap to close a chronic oroantral fistula. The effect is localized and is less marked with time. In this case it did not interfere with denture wearing

occasionally a combination of the two flaps might be necessary to close large defects but this has the disadvantage of placing the suture line over the defect and not on sound bone.

The buccal advancement flap technique has been criticized because of the postoperative decrease in sulcus depth (Figure 5.11). However, according to Eneroth and Martensson (1961), follow-up studies carried out by Schrudde at Rehrmann's clinic showed this to be only a temporary problem. He studied models produced from alginate impressions of the sulcus before and after operation and showed that the decrease in depth present at 2 weeks had disappeared after about 8 weeks.

The palatal rotation flap provides a thick layer of mucoperiosteum with a rich blood supply to support the clot. However, it has two main disadvantages: the folded palatal tissue may remain thick and bulky at the point of rotation of the flap; and there is denuded palatal bone present postoperatively.

Buccal advancement flap: operative technique (Figure 5.12)

1. Anaesthesia is secured with generous buccal and palatal infiltrations (Figure 5.12a).
2. The epithelial lining of the fistula is excised with a pointed no. 11 blade, using a circular cut into the depth of the fistula (Figure 5.12b). This is particularly important in a chronic oroantral fistula.
3. Two buccal incisions down to bone diverge from the attached gingival margin into the depth of the buccal sulcus (Figure 5.12c).
4. The trapezoid flap is raised off the underlying bone with a periosteal elevator (Figure 5.12d,e). The flap will not stretch over the defect because of the inelastic periosteum (Figure 5.12f).
5. The periosteum is divided by cutting through that layer alone, on the undersurface of the flap parallel to the base (Figure 5.12g). This allows the flap to lengthen and to be fitted to the palatal side of the fistula without tension (Figure 5.12h,i). Any tension on the flap suggests that the periosteum has not been adequately divided and often the anterior and posterior margins require further incision.

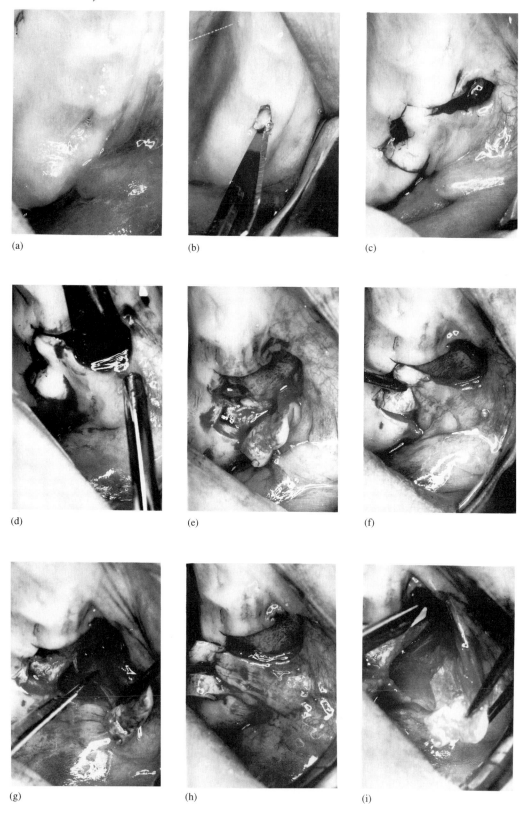

(a)

(b)

(c)

(d)

(e)

(f)

(g)

(h)

(i)

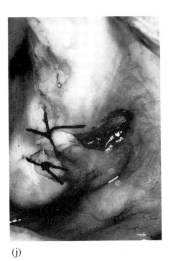

(j)

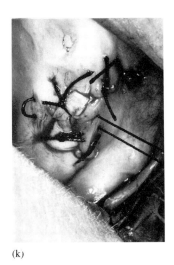

(k)

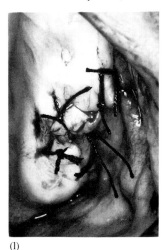

(l)

Figure 5.12 (a)–(l) Sequence of photographs illustrating the closure of a chronic oroantral fistula under local anaesthesia. Each stage is described in the text. From McGowan (1989)

6. The palatal tissue immediately surrounding the fistula is elevated slightly off the bone to facilitate suturing.
7. The flap is sutured in place using a combination of interrupted and horizontal mattress sutures (Figure 5.12j,k). Interrupted sutures can be used throughout but horizontal mattress sutures are useful in supporting the flap in broad apposition (Figure 5.12k,l). If the ends of the mattress sutures are cut longer, they are easier to distinguish at the time of removal (Figure 5.14l).

Palatal rotation flap: operative technique (Figure 5.13)

The palatal flap is a rotation flap based on the greater palatine artery (Figure 5.13a).

1. Adequate analgesia is obtained. The incisive branch of the nasopalatine nerve as well as the greater palatine nerve may need to be blocked. Buccal infiltration is also required.
2. It is important to ensure that the flap is made long enough to permit its rotation on to sound buccal bone. The flap is incised through mucoperiosteum down to bone and elevated with a Howarth's or Ward's periosteal elevator (Figure 5.13b).
3. The fistulous tract is excised with a triangular no. 11 blade.
4. The palatal flap is rotated to cover the oroantral fistula (Figure 5.13c). Care must be taken not to twist the flap too acutely as this may reduce the blood supply. A small V may be cut into the lateral side of the flap, lateral to the greater palatine artery, to make the rotated flap less bulky.
5. The flap is sutured in position with 3/0 silk interrupted and horizontal mattress sutures.
6. The denuded palatal bone is covered with ribbon gauze, soaked in Whitehead's varnish and sutured over the defect. It is left until the bone is covered in granulation tissue by approximately 14 days. Periodontal packing material may be used instead, and can be applied in a prefabricated acrylic vacuum-formed splint which has been generously relieved.

Figure 5.13 (a)–(c) The palatal
rotation flap technique

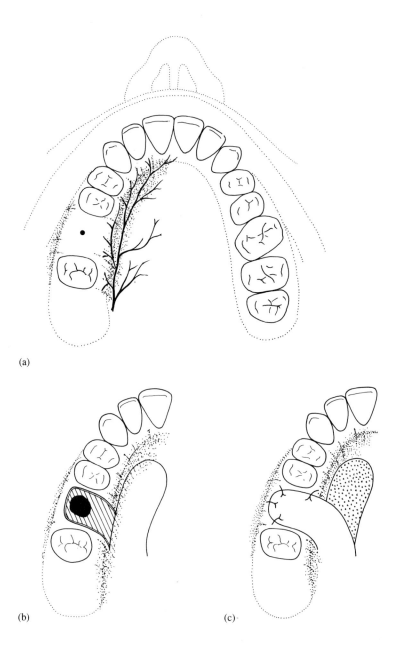

(a)

(b)   (c)

Postoperative care

Whichever surgical approach has been used, the patient should be advised to
avoid nose blowing and to keep the wound clean using warm saline mouthwashes
and by brushing adjacent areas with a toothbrush.

Amoxycillin 500 mg orally, steam inhalations, and ephedrine nasal drops 0.5%
via the nostril of the affected side should be administered three times daily for 5
days. In cases of penicillin allergy, erythromycin 250 mg four times daily for 5
days is a useful alternative. The inhalations and nasal drops may be continued for
a few more days if the sinus is not draining freely.

The sutures are removed 7 – 10 days after surgery, when there should be no evidence of fistula. Breakdown at this stage usually means the procedure has to be repeated. However, spontaneous closure can still be hoped for, and further surgery should be delayed for at least 4 weeks. It may be worth providing a simple acrylic plate to cover the defect during this time to prevent food being pushed into the antrum.

Root in antrum

The inadvertent displacement of a root or even a whole tooth into the maxillary sinus may complicate the creation of an oroantral fistula.

Following incomplete extraction of a tooth, the apical segment remaining in the socket may be dislodged by injudicious use of elevators, either into the antrum or beneath the palatal or buccal mucosa. Displacement of a premolar tooth into the antrum has been reported following the use of a mouth gag during general anaesthesia (Critchlow, 1975) and unerupted third molars are sometimes displaced into it by injudicious elevation. Lee (1978) found that the roots of the upper first molar were most often displaced and the palatal root accounted for 76% of these (Figure 5.16).

Historical

The earliest published report of a root dislodged into the maxillary sinus may be that of 'Mr. W.A.N. Cattlin, F.R.C.S. and L.D.S. of Islington'. A brief account of the case appears as part of a paper on 'Peculiarities of the interior of the antrum' read to the North London Medical Society and published in both the *British Medical Journal* of 12th June and the *Lancet* of 19th June 1858 (Cattlin, 1858a,b). It read as follows:

> The fang of a tooth had, during an attempt to extract it, passed completely into the antrum. The patient being a gentleman whose father had died of secondary malignant disease of the jaw, a consultation was held with an eminent hospital surgeon, and it was thought advisable under the circumstances to trephine the antrum; but although two large openings were made, and the cavity was frequently explored and injected, at the expiration of an hour's search, three surgeons had failed to remove the fang. On the second day a large quantity of water was forcibly injected from a powerful enema syringe, but with no better success; and on the third day Mr. Cattlin constructed a small gutta-percha scoop, which was attached to the end of a gold probe bent at such angles as to sweep the floor of any pocket in which the foreign body might have lodged. With the aid of this simple instrument (which was exhibited) the fang was readily removed in the course of a few seconds. It was somewhat surprising that so little pain followed from the operation and the irritation of the lining membrane. After two or three days the patient pursued his ordinary business, and at the end of three months the parts looked perfectly healthy, and had apparently filled up with bone. A small quantity of healthy mucus could, however, be forced through a very minute opening in the gum about four months after the operation; but very little inconvenience of any kind was suffered after the first two days.

A fuller account of this case had been presented at a monthly meeting of the Odontological Society of London in February 1858 and appears in their published Proceedings. As always in these old accounts, one has as much admiration for the fortitude of the patient as for the skill of the surgeon. The indication for removal of the 'fang' in this case is interesting and implies that the accident was not unknown but that removal of dislodged roots was not usually attempted. Cattlin's 'scoop' has not survived but his collection of specimens of maxillae illustrating his lecture is now preserved in the Odontological Museum of the Royal College of Surgeons of England and some have been photographed to illustrate this book (see Figure 1.6 and 1.11).

Diagnosis

When displacement is suspected, careful inspection with the aid of well-directed light and a fine suction tip and palpation of the socket area should be carried out to make sure that the root is not still in the socket or beneath the buccal or palatal mucosa. A periapical or occlusal radiograph will usually show a root within the sinus just above the extraction socket (Figures 5.14–5.16). A break in the continuity of the floor of the antrum shows the point of entry (Figure 5.17). The presence of a root canal confirms that the opacity is a retained root fragment (Figure 5.15, 5.16). A panoramic radiograph is a useful additional view if the root is not visible on intraoral films because it proves a clearer view of the sinus floor. An occipitomental view records the appearance of the sinus, which is helpful for both clinical and medicolegal reasons (Figure 5.18) and may also show the displaced root.

It is preferable to remove the root promptly to reduce the chances of producing a chronic maxillary sinusitis. There is also the possibility of discharge of a root through the antronasal duct into the nose and its inhalation. Sims (1985) reports a case in which a root 'migrated' through the antrum following its displacement

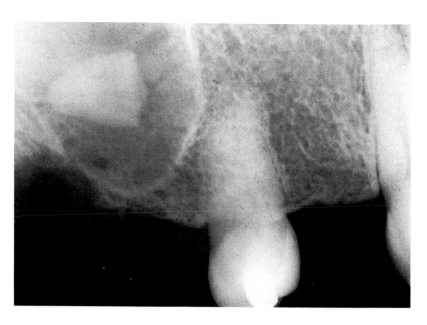

Figure 5.14 Root displaced into the right maxillary sinus by attempted elevation

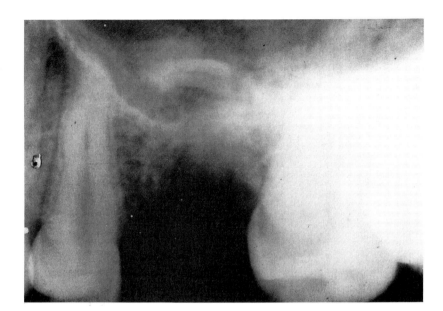

Figure 5.15 Molar root fractured during first molar extraction and displaced into the adjacent sinus

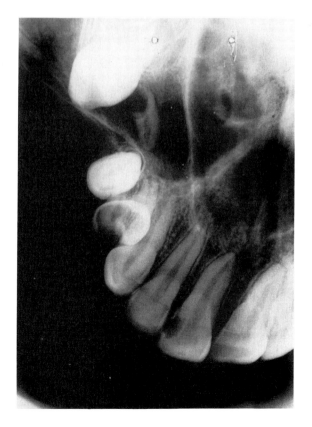

Figure 5.16 Occlusal radiograph of a root displaced into the sinus. The wider view is helpful if the root has been displaced away from the socket

Figure 5.17 Panoramic radiograph which shows a root displaced into the right maxillary sinus and lying anterior to the socket

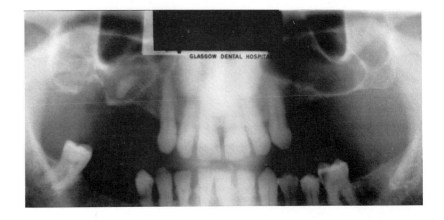

Figure 5.18 A root has been displaced into the left maxillary sinus but the 'cloudiness' of the sinuses is due to pre-existing disease and not to infection caused by the accident

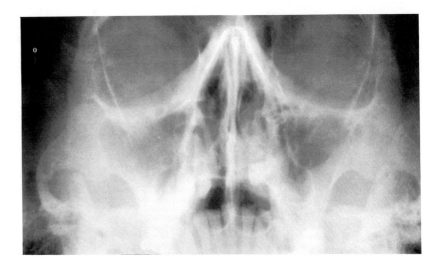

and became lodged in the ostium. Killey and Kay (1964) reported five cases where roots displaced into the antrum were expelled from the nose during sneezing and coughing attacks.

Surgical removal

There are two surgical approaches to the root, either through the site of the tooth socket or through the canine fossa by the so-called Caldwell–Luc approach. Because of the tapering shape of the surface of the maxilla the approaches converge and the part of the facial wall of the sinus which is removed for access is similar (Figure 5.19).

It is essential when using either approach that a radiograph is taken immediately before surgery as a mobile root may be difficult to find. A good light source and efficient surgical suction apparatus are also absolute requirements. Occasionally the root can be retrieved using the suction tip alone, but more often it has to be visualized and then grasped with suitable forceps.

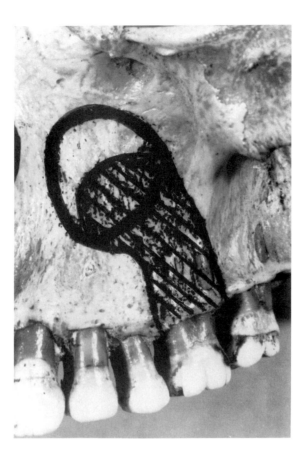

Figure 5.19 The areas of bone removal for the canine fossa (Caldwell–Luc) approach and the socket approach to the sinus for removal of a displaced root. The socket approach area is hatched and the alternatives can be seen to overlap considerably

Removal through the tooth socket

If the root is near to the extraction socket and a fistula is present, this is the method of choice because it allows retrieval of the root and closure of the fistula at the same operation (Figure 5.20). A buccal flap is raised and bone is removed from the buccal wall of the extraction socket to create a window into the antrum above it. Careful suction clears the antrum of blood clot and the root is located and retrieved using non-toothed forceps (Fickling's pattern are ideal), taking care to avoid its further displacement into the antrum. The sinus is irrigated with normal saline and the buccal flap advanced to close the fistula.

Antibiotics, nasal drops and inhalations are prescribed as described above for oroantral fistula closure. Healing is usually uneventful, without the need for any further treatment.

Caldwell–Luc Approach (Figure 5.21)

An incision is made in the buccal sulcus from the lateral incisor to the first molar and can be extended if required. The mucoperiostal flap is raised and retracted and an opening made into the sinus through the thin bone of the canine fossa.

Figure 5.20 (a)–(f) A sequence of photographs showing removal of a recently fractured root of an upper molar tooth from the sinus through the socket

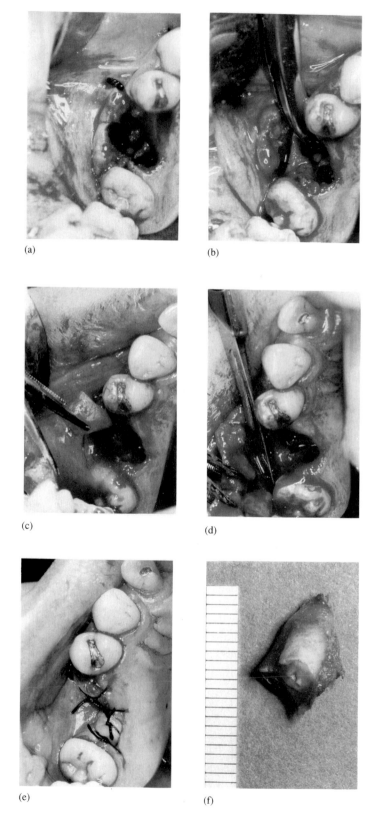

(a)

(b)

(c)

(d)

(e)

(f)

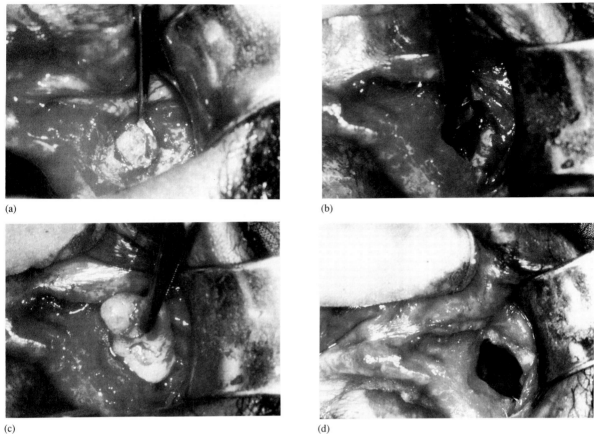

(a)

(b)

(c)

(d)

Figure 5.21 (a)–(d) A sequence of photographs showing the removal a displaced molar tooth from the left maxillary sinus of an otherwise edentulous patient via the canine fossa

Any blood or granulation tissue must be carefully removed using a sucker and curved or angled artery forceps. The radiograph taken immediately before surgery indicates the area in which the root will be located. This approach provides good access but if the root has not penetrated the antral mucosa and lies between it and the bone, then it may be not be visible. Large root fragments are not difficult to find but if the root has been present in the sinus for some time it may be covered in granulation tissue or a fibrous scar. Following retrieval with curved artery forceps or the sucker tip, areas of oedematous lining or polyps may be removed and the sinus irrigated with normal saline. The incision is closed with interrupted 3/0 black silk sutures.

Antibiotics, nasal drops and inhalations are prescribed as for an oroantral fistula and the non-absorbable sutures are removed after 7–10 days.

Other foreign bodies

Rahman (1982) reported the removal of fine matchsticks from the maxillary sinus of a patient who had used them to apply salt on cottonwool in a vain attempt to produce closure of a small oroantral fistula. Bullets or missile fragments may come to lodge in the sinus in war, or accidental injury (O'Connell and Pahor, 1991), and part of a more ancient weapon, the tip of a wooden spear, was removed from the maxillary sinus of a young man in Papua, New Guinea, by Gupta, Murthy and Pulotu (1990).

Fractures

Fractured tuberosity

This occurs most frequently when extracting a lone-standing upper third molar (Figure 5.22). If the bone is found to be moving with the tooth during extraction, the operator should stop immediately (Figure 5.23). Continued application of extraction force can lead to removal of the surrounding bone, adjacent teeth, mucosa and tuberosity, in addition to the tooth. The loss of mucosa is particularly damaging as it is unavailable for closure of the defect.

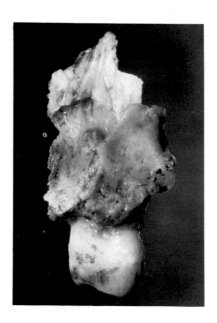

Figure 5.22 Tuberosity which has been fractured during extraction of the third molar and removed. The bone at the top of the specimen is paper thin and translucent.

Figure 5.23 (a) Buccal and (b) palatal views of a fractured tuberosity caused by the attempted extraction of an upper left molar. Unfortunately, the gingival soft tissues have been severely lacerated both buccally and palatally and this created difficulty in opposing flaps when the loose tooth and attached bone were removed

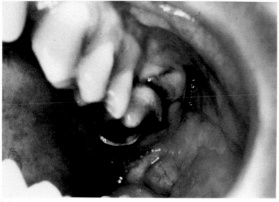

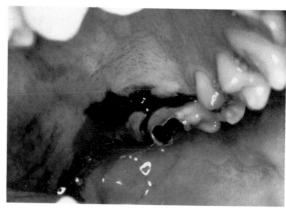

(a)   (b)

It may be easier to leave the tooth in place and allow the fracture to heal before making a further attempt to remove it (Figure 5.24). The tuberosity should be retained to help with denture retention (Figure 5.25). Surgical removal from healed intact bone is considerably easier than removing the tooth from mobile bone, which may itself be difficult to retain. The fracture should be immobilized to promote healing but if there are no functional opposing teeth splinting is unnecessary and the patient should simply try to chew on the opposite side. Where there are opposing teeth and other teeth in the same arch, a splint can be constructed to immobilize the fragment in the correct position, or an upper arch bar, which is rigid enough to prevent displacement, can be used.

If pain is the reason for the extraction, this pain must be relieved. Immediate removal of the tooth is indicated unless the pulp chamber can be opened for pulp extirpation or drainage of a pulpal or periapical abscess. The extent of the fracture is determined by gently moving the involved tooth from side to side while observing and then palpating the surrounding tissues. If only a small fragment of bone is involved, the tooth should be removed immediately. If pain is not the reason for extracting the tooth, and other teeth or a large amount of bone are involved, the fracture should be allowed to heal before proceeding.

When a flap has been raised to remove a fractured tuberosity, the fracture is often found to be more extensive than anticipated, but providing the bone is not

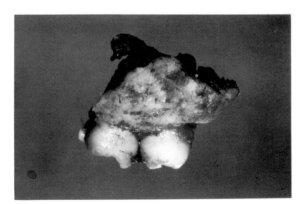

Figure 5.24 A fractured tuberosity carrying the two last molar teeth. Removal of the posterior tooth first might have avoided the problem

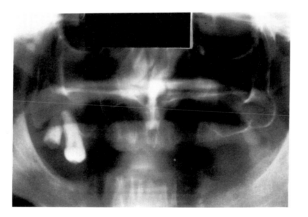

Figure 5.25 Panoramic radiograph of a patient otherwise successfully rendered edentulous whose right tuberosity has been fractured; again, extraction of the posterior carious root first would have been wiser

grossly mobile, and has not been completely stripped of its periosteum, the fragment can be retained and the fracture should heal. The tooth is sectioned using a bur, and the pieces carefully removed. If the fracture is very mobile and the survival of the bone doubtful, it has to be removed *en bloc* with the tooth (Figures 5.22 and 5.24). The flap raised should therefore be sufficiently large to allow removal of the fragment without tearing the mucosa. Any relieving limbs of the incision should be planned to lie on sound bone following removal of the fractured portion.

If it is decided to delay tooth removal until after splinting and healing of the fracture, the tooth has then to be sectioned and surgically removed with great delicacy. The healed bone remains weak and attempted forceps extraction can recreate the original problem.

Tuberosity fracture inevitably involves the maxillary sinus. Antibiotics, nasal drops and inhalations are therefore prescribed to help prevent development of a chronic oroantral fistula.

Other fractures involving the maxillary sinus

Fractures involving the maxillary sinus are those of the zygomatic complex, Le Fort I, II and III fractures and orbital floor blow-out fractures. The Le Fort classification (Le Fort, 1901) was devised to bring order to the chaos described by Hamilton (1860): 'These fractures assume so great a variety in respect to form, situation and complications, that it would be impossible to speak of them symptomatically or to establish anything but very general rules as to treatment and prognosis.' These comments emphasize the variable fracture patterns which occur and the necessity of considering the fragments as composite blocks of bone. Reduction and fixation of Le Fort fractures is usually performed within 24–48 hours of injury, whereas zygomatic complex and orbital floor fractures may be easier to treat after 5 days, when the bruising and swelling has subsided.

Zygomatic complex

Assaults often result in fracture of the zygomatic complex. The fractures occur at lines of weakness and pass through the orbital floor, usually medial to the zygomaticomaxillary suture, and therefore inevitably involve the sinus. Whether there is only mild displacement or considerable disruption, the fractured zygoma is forced into the sinus, which lies beneath it.

The main indications for treatment are diplopia on upward gaze, restriction of mandibular movements, especially lateral excursion towards the fractured side, infraorbital nerve anaesthesia which does not resolve, or a cosmetic defect caused by the loss of malar prominence, which is best visualized from above.

There may also be unilateral epistaxis and subconjunctival haemorrhage laterally with no posterior limit. If there is a marked orbital defect, symptoms associated with this will be evident (see below).

Radiographs   Occipitomental views are the most helpful in diagnosing a fracture of the zygomatic complex (Figure 5.26). The malar bone should be visualized as a four-pointed star, each point of the star representing an area where

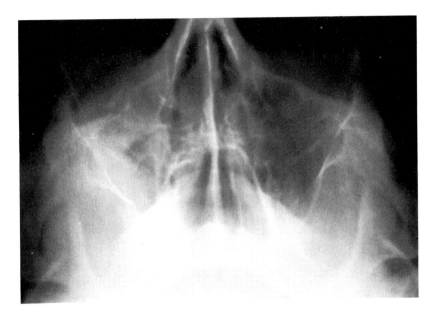

Figure 5.26 Occipitomental radiograph of a patient with a fracture of the right zygoma. The sinuses are asymmetrical and the right is cloudy due to contained blood. The fractured bones are seen at the zygomaticofrontal suture, the lower lateral sinus wall and the infraorbital rim, where a small separate fragment can be seen close to the right infraorbital foramen. The fourth point of fracture of the zygomatic arch is not visible on this view

fracture occurs. There will be varying displacement at each site and there may be comminution of the bone, depending on the force of injury. Opacity or a fluid level in the maxillary sinus is due to pooling of blood and this produces unilateral epistaxis as it escapes from the sinus via the antronasal duct.

Treatment   Simply elevating the malar via the Gillies temporal approach may suffice, but if the malar is unstable fixation is required. This may be achieved by transosseous wiring or plating at the lines of fracture, extraoral pinning, or support by an antral pack of ribbon gauze soaked in Whitehead's varnish.

Finlay, Ward-Booth and Moos (1984) have shown that antral packing is associated with a higher incidence of postoperative sinusitis than other methods. If it is to be used, packing must be performed carefully after all bony manipulation is complete in order to avoid impingement of sharp bony spicules on to the ophthalmic artery, producing spasm and retinal ischaemia which results in blindness.

Any foreign material within the sinus should be removed via a Caldwell–Luc opening. Even though there may be considerable comminution of the anterolateral and posterolateral walls of the antrum they do not require exploration because they heal satisfactorily without intervention.

Le Fort I fracture

This low-level fracture splits the dentoalveolar portion from the rest of the maxilla. It is an extension of the fractured tuberosity and can occur unilaterally with a palatal split, or bilaterally. There may be very little displacement and in the edentulous patient it may not require active treatment. On the other hand, there can be marked displacement and impaction of the maxilla.

Mobility of the maxilla is detected clinically by palpation above the apices of the upper anterior teeth while pressure is placed upon the crowns of these teeth in an anteroposterior direction. A 'cracked cup' sound is elicited when the teeth are percussed and if the fractured segment is displaced there will be derangement of the occlusion. Lateral radiographs show the line of fracture passing just above the floor of the antrum.

Treatment, as in any fracture, consists of reduction and immobilization. The maxillary fracture may be reduced with finger pressure or using a set of Rowe's disimpaction forceps. The straight blade of the forceps (right or left) is placed below the inferior turbinate along the floor of the nose and the rounded blade is placed in the palate. The fracture is reduced until there is no step palpable at the fracture site. After removal of the forceps the occlusion can be checked.

Unilateral fractures can be fixed to the opposite side of the maxilla using cast cap splints or an arch bar. In bilateral fractures the maxilla can be immobilized by 'suspending' it from above with circumzygomatic wires. If the zygomatic complex is also fractured, frontal suspension wires passing from the zygomatic process of the frontal bone medial to the zygomatic arch will be needed.

Extensive interdigitation of the teeth and secure intermaxillary fixation are needed to prevent these methods of fixation pulling the maxilla backwards. The Levant frame fixes the maxilla extraorally to supraorbital pins and produces a forward pull on the maxilla. Internal fixation with miniplates provides rigid immobilization.

The maxilla is usually stable at 4–5 weeks, when fixation can be removed.

Le Fort II fracture (Figure 5.27)

This is a higher level 'pyramidal' fracture of the mid-face. Unlike the Le Fort I fracture, where facial swelling may be minimal, the soft tissues tend to 'balloon' due to oedema and ecchymosis. As with the Le Fort III fracture, this may produce the classical bilateral 'black eyes'. A palpating finger placed on the infraorbital

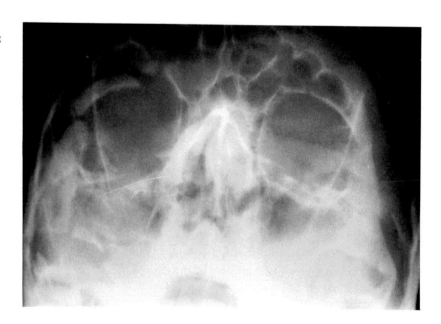

Figure 5.27 Radiograph of a complex Le Fort II fracture showing disruption of the outlines of the orbits and opacity of the maxillary sinuses

rims may detect movement here when pressure is applied to the upper anterior teeth.

Treatment is as for a Le Fort I fracture: repositioning and immobilization to a stable part of the facial skeleton.

Le Fort III fracture

This is at a higher level still than the Le Fort II fracture and causes complete dislocation of the facial skeleton from the cranial base. Theoretically the maxillary sinuses would be unaffected .but in practice the degree of injury is usually so severe as to produce a complex pattern of multiple fracture lines, some of which will involve these sinuses.

The clinical presentation is of a similar but more severe injury than the Le Fort II fracture. The nose is filled with blood, and backward displacement of the maxilla can compromise the airway. The face may appear longer with 'hooding' of the eyes, and there will be cerebrospinal fluid rhinorrhoea. When pressure is applied to the upper anterior dentoalveolar segment, movement may be palpated at the frontozygomatic and frontonasal sutures.

Many middle-third fractures are complicated combinations and asymmetric variations of the basic patterns described.

Complications of fractures involving the maxillary sinus

It is not usual to explore the sinus at the same time as fixation of the fracture unless the presence of a foreign body is suspected. Despite the often gross comminution of the sinus walls, little sinus pathology seems to result. Kreidler and Koch (1975) found endoscopic evidence of chronic inflammatory mucosal changes in 35% of patients 7 years after fixation of maxillary fractures without sinus exploration, but all patients were asymptomatic and primary sinus surgery was not indicated. The figure of 35% should be set against the 46% of a group of uninjured patients surveyed radiographically by Wilson and Grocutt (1990). Of 45 patients who sustained Le Fort I, II and III fractures and where only comminuted open sinus fractures were explored, a single case of post-traumatic sinusitis was observed in a follow-up period of 6 months to 6 years (Heimgartner-Candinas, Heimgartner and Jonutis, 1978).

Orbital floor blow-out fractures

The orbital floor may be breached as part of a middle-third fracture, but isolated blow-out fractures of the orbital floor also occur.

The orbital cavity is cone shaped and sudden pressure on the globe from an object such as a tennis or squash ball pushes the orbital contents backwards into the smaller part of the orbit. The rapid increase in intraorbital pressure is transmitted to the orbital walls and fracture occurs at the thinnest parts.

Loss of the continuity of the orbital floor allows herniation of periorbital fat and extravasated blood from the ruptured periosteum into the maxillary sinus. This produces the typical 'hanging drop' radiographic appearance (Figure 5.28). The inferior oblique and the inferior rectus muscles may also be tethered, as evidenced by persistent diplopia on upward and outward or upward gaze (Figure 5.29), and confirmed by the forced duction test. The patient may also have

Figure 5.28 (a) Occipitomental and (b) tomographic views of a blow-out fracture of the left orbit; the 'hanging drop' appearance is clearly seen

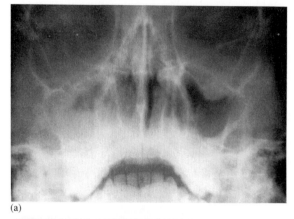

(a)

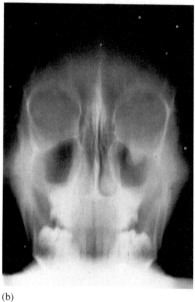

(b)

Figure 5.29 Impaired movement of the left eye causing diplopia in the patient whose radiographs are seen above (5.28 (a) and (b)). She is attempting to look upwards and to the left. There had been no treatment at the time of injury

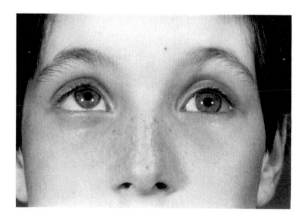

periorbital oedema and ecchymosis in the early stages, enophthalmos with or without apparent ptosis, and infraorbital nerve damage.

Radiographs should be taken to confirm the diagnosis, the most useful being tomograms taken at varying depths of cut or CT scans. In addition to the 'hanging drop', other features which may be seen are orbital emphysema and an opaque antrum. Objective assessment and monitoring of the interference with ocular function is essential (Al-Qurainy *et al.*, 1991).

Treatment involves retrieving the orbital contents from the antrum and repairing the orbital floor defect. The approach to the orbital floor is via an infraorbital or a blepharoplasty incision, giving a direct view of the orbital floor. The displaced tissues are carefully retrieved from the maxillary sinus and a sheet of Silastic material or bone is used to reconstruct the orbital floor.

Late treatment of orbital floor blow-out fractures is unsatisfactory because extensive fibrous scarring and periorbital tissue atrophy leave a residual combination of enophthalmos and limitation of ocular movements which is very difficult to correct.

Pneumocele and cheek emphysema

A pneumocele of the orbit occurs following forceful blowing of the nose when there is a small bony defect in the roof of the sinus. The patient should be given antibiotics and observed for developing orbital cellulitis. Onset of sluggish pupillary reaction to light and accommodation are signs of optic nerve swelling and mean that urgent surgical decompression is required to prevent blindness.

Air emphysema of the cheek also may follow fracture of the facial wall of the sinus which can be associated with trauma to the inferior orbital rim.

Orthognathic surgery

Le Fort I osteotomies are carried out for the correction of various types of maxillary deformity and involve bone cuts directly into the maxillary sinuses with down-fracture of the maxilla (Figure 5.30).

Despite this direct surgical trauma to the antral lining and presumed disturbance of the physiological clearing mechanism of the sinus, infections are rare when antibiotics are used. In a series of more than 200 patients who underwent a Le Fort I procedure for vertical maxillary excess (Bell, Thrash and Zysset 1986), only two developed a clinical infection and one of these did not take any medication after surgery. Radiographically, the air–fluid level is no longer visible after 2–4 weeks and the mucosal reaction gradually diminishes.

Epker and Woolford (1975) consider that the sinuses should be evaluated before Le Fort II and III osteomies because preoperative sinus disease leads to increased sinus problems postoperatively. Resolution of pre-existing chronic sinus disease by conservative or surgical treatment should be included in the preparation of these patients for surgery. Where there was no sinus disease present before surgery, these authors found that none occurred postoperatively.

Figure 5.30 Two views of a down-fractured maxilla during an operation to correct maxillomandibular dysharmony. A collection of blood can be seen pooling in the otherwise healthy right and left sinuses in (a), and the separated floor of the sinuses is displayed in (b)

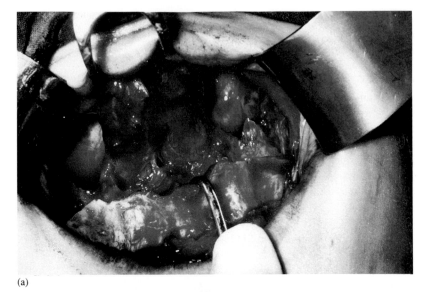

(a)

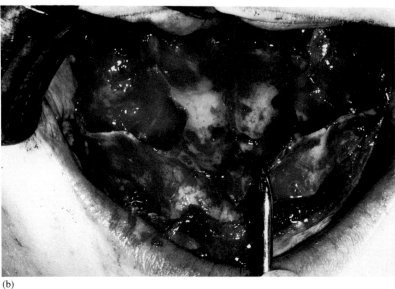

(b)

References

Al-Qurainy, I. A., Titterington, D. M., Dutton, G. N., Stassen, L. F. A., Moos, K. F. and El-Attar, A. (1991) Midfacial fractures and the eye: the development of a system for detecting patients at risk of eye injury. *British Journal of Oral and Maxillofacial Surgery*, **29**, 363–367

Bell, C. S., Thrash, W. J. and Zysset, M. K. (1986) Incidence of maxillary sinusitis following Le Fort I maxillary osteotomy. *Journal of Oral and Maxillofacial Surgery*. **44**, 100–103

Cattlin, W. A. N. (1858a) Untitled. *Transactions of the Odontological Society of London 1857–1860*, **2**, 15

Cattlin, W. A. N. (1858b) Peculiarities of the interior of the antrum; case in which a fang of a tooth was impacted in a pocket of the antrum. *BMJ*, **12th June**, 485; *Lancet*, **17th June**, 614

Critchlow, H. A. (1975) Injury to the antrum from use of mouth gag. *British Dental Journal*, **139**, 406

Ehrl, P. A. (1980) Oroantral communication. *International Journal of Oral Surgery*, **9**, 351–358

Eneroth, C. M. and Mårtenssøn, G. (1961) Closure of antro-alveolar fistulae. *Acta Oto-laryngologica*, (Stockholm) **53**, 477–485

Epker, B. N. and Woolford, L. M. (1975) Middle third facial osteotomies: their use in the correction of acquired and developmental dentofacial and craniofacial deformities. *Journal of Oral Surgery*, **33**, 491–514

Finlay, P. M., Ward-Booth, R. P. and Moos, K. F. (1984) Morbidity associated with the use of antral packs and external pins in the treatment of unstable fracture of the zygomatic complex. *British Journal of Oral and Maxillofacial Surgery*, **22**, 18–23

Gupta, A. C., Murthy, D. P. and Pulotu, M. L. (1990) Unusual type of foreign body in the maxillary sinus. *Journal of Laryngology and Otology*, **104**, 718–719

Hamilton, F. H. (1860) *Practical Treatise on Fractures and Dislocations*. Blanchard and Lea, Philadelphia

Heimgartner-Candinas, B., Heimgartner, M. and Jonutis, A. (1978) Results of treatment of midfacial fractures. Indications for exploration and drainage of the maxillary sinuses. *Journal of Maxillofacial Surgery*, **6**, 293–301

Killey, H. C. and Kay, L. W. (1964) Possible sequelae when a tooth or root is dislodged into the maxillary sinus. *British Dental Journal*, **116**, 73–77

Kreidler, J. F. and Koch, H. (1975) Endoscopic findings of maxillary sinus after middle face fractures. *Journal of Maxillofacial Surgery*, **3**, 10–14

Lee, F. M. S. (1978) Management of the displaced root in the maxillary sinus. *International Journal of Oral Surgery*, **7**, 374–379

Le Fort, R. (1901) Etude experimentale sur les fractures de la machoire superieure. *Revue de Chirurgie*, **23**, 208–227, 360–379, 479–507

Lund, V. J. (1986) The design and function of intranasal antrostomies. *Journal of Laryngology and Otology*, **100**, 35–39

McGowan, D. A. (1989) *An Atlas of Minor Oral Surgery*, Dunitz, London, chap. 12

Mitchell, R. and Lamb, J. (1983) Immediate closure of oro-antral communications with a collagen implant. A preliminary report. *British Dental Journal*, **154**, 171–174

O'Connell, J. and Pahor, A. L. (1991) Untitled report. *BMJ*, **302**, 1476

Rahman, A. (1982) Foreign bodies in the maxillary sinus. *British Dental Journal*, **153**, 308.

Rehrmann, A. (1936) Eine methode zur Schliessung von Kieferhöhle-Perforationen. *Deutsche Zahnärztliche Wochenschrift*, **39**, 1136–1138

Sims, A. P. T. (1985) A dental root in the ostium of the maxillary antrum. *British Journal of Oral and Maxillofacial Surgery*, **23**, 67–73

Von Wowern, N. (1970) Frequency of oro-antral fistulae after perforation to the maxillary sinus. *Scandinavian Journal of Dental Research*, **78**, 394–396

Wilson, P. S. and Grocutt, M. (1990) Mucosal thickening on sinus x-ray and its significance. *Journal of Laryngology and Otology*, **104**, 694 –695

Chapter 6

Malignant disease

As the maxillary sinus is a closed and concealed site, neoplasms within it can reach a considerable size before signs or symptoms develop. The consequent delay in diagnosis is largely responsible for the poor prognosis of malignant disease of the area.

Spontaneous paraesthesia over any part of the face is an ominous finding and, in the middle third, malignant disease of the antrum or nasopharynx is the most likely cause. A chronic sinusitis, particularly if unilateral, which does not respond to treatment, or epistaxis in a non-hypertensive patient over the age of 40 years, should be regarded as suggestive of an underlying malignancy.

Any dental pain, localized or referred, or teeth with unexplained mobility should be thoroughly investigated. The increasing use of the orthopantomogram for dental diagnostic screening purposes offers an opportunity for routine examination of the maxillary sinuses, and it is important to be aware of the radiological features of antral malignancy. It can only be hoped that more frequent early diagnosis will lead to a more favourable prognosis for these tumours.

Incidence

Carcinoma of any paranasal sinus is rare and accounts for about 0.2–0.8% of all malignancies (Batsakis, 1979), with 80% of lesions arising in the maxillary sinus (Harrison, 1971). These form 7% of head and neck cancers if the eye, brain and peripheral nervous system are excluded (Hole, 1991). Figures based on the years 1985–1989 for the West of Scotland (population about 2 million) record an average of six cases per annum of paranasal sinus carcinoma, of which about a third were maxillary sinus cancers (West of Scotland Cancer Surveillance Unit, personal communication 1991). One possible reason for the difference in proportion of paranasal sinus tumours in different series is that the initial site is difficult to determine when the tumour involves several different sinuses at presentation.

In their study of South African Blacks, who have the highest known incidence of jaw cancer in the world, Higginson and Oettle (1960) found that all carcinomas of the paranasal sinuses arose within the maxillary antra. They represented 1.7–3.4% of all male malignancy and 0–2.8% of all female cancers. The lower figures related to city dwellers, the higher to the rural population. These cancers are approximately twice as common in men as women and nearly 95% of patients are over 40 years of age (Batsakis, 1979).

Of the malignant neoplasms arising from the maxillary sinus, 80% are squamous cell carcinomas. Adenocarcinomas and undifferentiated carcinomas are much less common. Of 23 carcinomas of the maxillary antrum examined histologically in the South African series, 70% were squamous carcinomas, 13% were transitional cell carcinomas, 13% were anaplastic and 4% were adenocarcinomas (Higginson and Oettle, 1960). Melanoma, neuroblastoma and sarcoma also occur, though even less frequently.

Melanoma arises from melanocytes which migrate from the neural crest to the maxillary sinus mucosa during embryonic development and the maxillary sinus is the site of 80% of paranasal sinus melanomas (Ramos, Som and Solodnik, 1990). Lymphoma may occur in association with more widespread disease but the maxillary sinus is a rare site for secondary tumour deposits.

Aetiology

Respiratory epithelium is known to undergo squamous metaplasia in the presence of infection and chronic sinusitis may therefore be a predisposing factor for antral carcinoma. In support of this view, Sakai, Shigematzu and Fuchihata (1972) in Japan found that 80% of maxillary carcinoma patients had a history of chronic sinusitis, and the chance of a person with this condition subsequently developing carcinoma of the sinus was 36 times greater than that of an unaffected individual.

Thorotrast was used as a contrast medium in radiological diagnosis in the late 1920s in Europe, particularly in Germany, Switzerland and Eastern France. One of its uses was to outline morphological changes in the sinuses. It is not excreted, has a long half-life (14 years), and decays to ten different radioactive daughter nuclides, so radioactivity from the decaying thorium-232 within Thorotrast takes about 30 years to reach its peak. Malignancy develops 12–24 years after exposure. In a review of the literature by Goren *et al.* (1980), 18 cases of malignant disease induced by this agent were identified.

Squamous carcinomas are more common in boot and shoe and in nickel workers (Barton, 1977). Adenocarcinomas of the nasal passages are an occupational hazard for furniture makers, and are also more common in footwear industry workers. This is assumed to be due to inhaled carcinogens in the dust produced during the manufacturing processes.

The use of indigenous snuff and the smoky atmosphere in their huts may be causal factors for carcinoma of the paranasal sinuses in the rural black South African population (Higginson and Oettle, 1960).

Signs and symptoms

A tumour confined to the sinus cavity is unlikely to become evident except as an incidental finding, unless it involves the infraorbital nerve and produces paraesthesia of the cheek, or erodes blood vessels, giving rise to epistaxis. Once the sinus walls are expanded or destroyed, symptoms arise from the involvement of neighbouring structures. The primary site and direction of spread govern the pattern of symptoms (Figure 6.1 and Table 6.1).

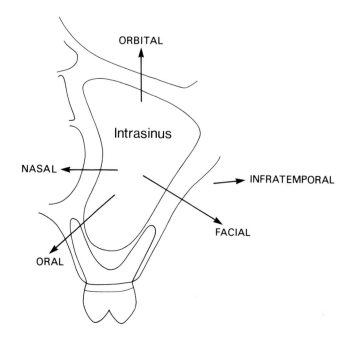

Figure 6.1 Diagram of the directions of tumour spread from the maxillary sinus

The relative frequency of presenting symptoms in published series inevitably reflects a degree of patient selection according to the speciality practised by the authors, but, unlike oral malignancies, dull pain seems to be a frequent symptom. This may be accounted for by the late presentation, the obstructive consequences of tissue bulk in the sinus cavity, and its almost inevitable infection.

In a series of 33 cases of maxillary sinus cancer, Mundy *et al.* (1985) found the most common symptoms were associated with the nose (33.8%) or the face (30.3%), with swelling being the most common (Figure 6.2a–c, 6.3b and 6.4). However, about a third of patients have oral symptoms including pain, and they may initially seek help from their dentist. Unexplained mobility of teeth or an

Table 6.1 Key symptoms of maxillary sinus malignant disease related to direction of tumour spread (Figure 6.1). Symptoms may be exacerbated by secondary infection

ORAL	Swelling
	Ulceration
	Mobility of teeth
NASAL	Obstruction
	Bloody discharge
	Epiphora
ORBITAL	Proptosis
	Diplopia
INFRATEMPORAL	Trismus
	Pain
FACIAL	Infraorbital paraesthesia
	Swelling
	Pain

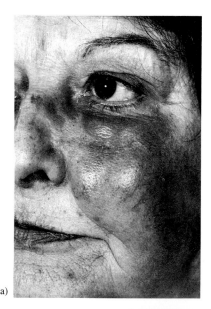

(a)

Figure 6.2 Patient presenting with an extensive carcinoma of the left maxillary sinus. (a) and (b) Photographs illustrating the cheek swelling and the elevated eye but only slight swelling of the palatal alveolus and in the buccal sulcus. (c) CT scan illustrating the obliteration of the sinus by tumour and the extensive bone destruction

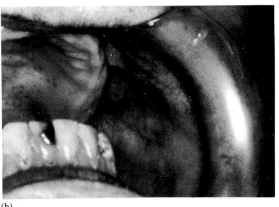

(b)

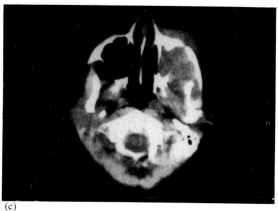

(c)

increasingly ill-fitting upper denture may be the first sign that a lesion is expanding intraorally. Extraction of a loose tooth may be followed by the appearance of tumour in the socket (see Figure 5.8). Palatal or alveolar ulceration is a late symptom (Figure 6.3).

Medial spread produces nasal obstruction and epistaxis and the tumour may be visible on nasal examination. Epiphora will result if the lacrimal sac or nasolacrimal duct is obstructed. Anterolateral extension produces facial swelling and paraesthesia and the submandibular lymph nodes may then be involved.

Invasion of the orbital contents initially increases their volume, producing proptosis and pushing the eye upwards, raising the pupillary level (Figure 6.4a). Later, direct involvement of nerves and muscles leads to diplopia, eye pain, visual loss, and eventually to facial pain and facial swelling. Posterior spread into the infratemporal fossa produces trismus by involvement of the pterygoid muscles (Figure 6.5). Paraesthesia of the mandibular nerve will also occur as the

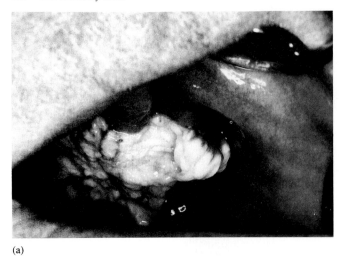

(a)

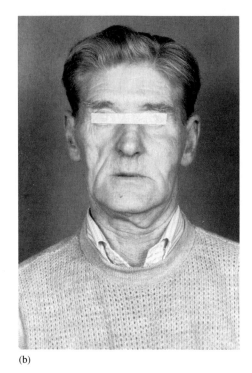

(b)

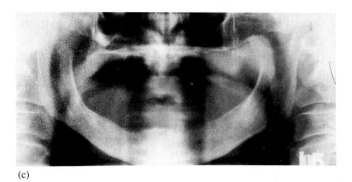

(c)

Figure 6.3 (a) Patient presenting with a large carcinoma of the left maxillary alveolar process. (b) There is some facial swelling, denoted by the partial obliteration of the left nasolabial fold, but no apparent orbital effects. Radiographs show (c) destruction of the alveolar bone; obliteration of the sinus by tumour; and (d) destruction of the lateral limit of the sinus wall. In contrast to the case illustrated in Figure 6.2, this lesion is likely to have originated in the mouth and spread to involve the sinus

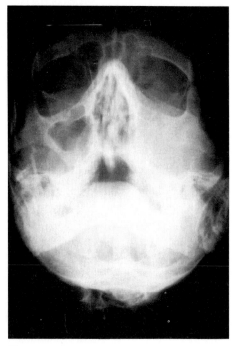

(d)

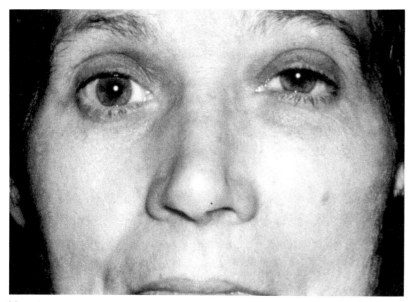

(a)

Figure 6.4 Patient with an advanced carcinoma of the left maxillary sinus showing elevation of the left eye. Facial swelling which has obliterated the nasolabial fold (a) is readily observed when examining the patient from above (b). Early mild swelling is best recognized this way

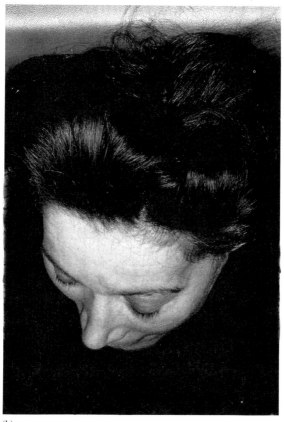

(b)

Figure 6.5 Invasion of the posterior part of the right maxillary sinus by a very extensive recurrent adenocarcinoma showing total destruction of the pterygoid plates

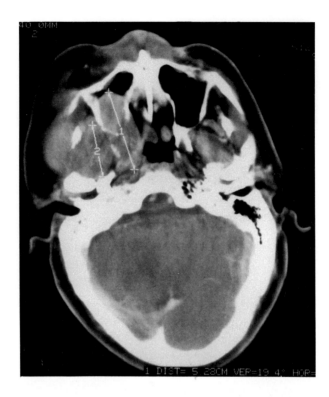

tumour invades towards the cranial base. Signs of spread to the pterygopalatine fossa, the infratemporal region and the base of skull are late and indicate a poor prognosis.

Spread to the regional lymph nodes is uncommon if the tumour is confined to the sinus. Because lymphatic drainage is firstly to the retropharyngeal nodes, which are not easily palpable, lympadenopathy is detected in only 15% of cases at presentation (Cheesman, 1987). Palpable lower deep cervical lymph nodes indicate advanced spread. Melanomas frequently involve the nose as well as the antrum at presentation and are seen as polypoid, highly vascular masses which commonly produce epistaxis and symptoms of nasal obstruction (Ramos, Som and Solodnik, 1990).

Any symptoms in the region of the maxillary sinus for which an obvious cause cannot be found should be regarded with suspicion and radiographs taken.

Radiology

An antral carcinoma may appear radiographically as a 'cloudy' antrum, a diffuse opacity or an irregular soft tissue outline. In advanced disease, bony erosion and destruction of the sinus walls may be evident.

The panoramic view of the jaws produced by rotational tomography defines the alveolar–sinus interface better than a Water's view (Figure 6.3c). However, most of the facial and posterolateral walls of the sinus are superimposed on the medial wall.

The occipitomental (Waters') view is most commonly used initially to search for evidence of malignant disease in the maxillary sinus (Figure 6.3d). Loss of the fine linear outline of the lateral wall is a particularly sensitive sign of bone destruction, but the posteroinferior part is obscured by the petrous temporal bone and the maxillary alveolar process and teeth. McGregor and McGregor (1986) state that radiographs may give false-negative results and that the actual extent of tumour is always greater than indicated on the radiographs.

Computed tomography (CT) has been an important advance in the radiological evaluation of malignant lesions of the maxillary sinus. Axial and coronal scans permit precise anatomical localization of tumour and more detailed preoperative planning of surgery or radiotherapy (Figure 6.6) Coronal scans obtained with the patient in the submentovertical position provide better information than coronal reconstructions from axial scans. Contrast enhancement may be helpful in assessing soft tissue involvement (Figure 6.6c). Erosion of bone, involvement of soft tissues, and posterosuperior extension into the orbit, pterygopalatine fossa

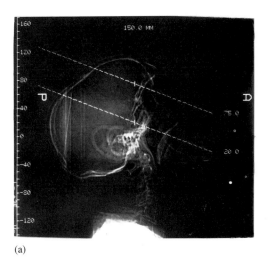

(a)

Figure 6.6 (a) Scout scans are used for precise orientation of the tomographic cuts in CT scanning. (b) The 'grey scale' of the scans can be adjusted, and (c) measurements made to help planning of surgery or radiotherapy

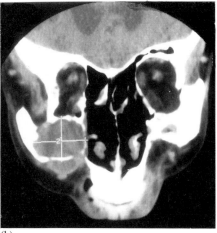

(b)

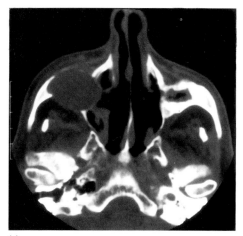

(c)

(Figure 6.5) and cranial cavity can be defined, allowing accurate planning of radiotherapy and surgery and estimation of the prognosis.

Magnetic resonance imaging (MRI) permits scanning in three planes and has the potential for accurate differentiation of invading tumour from a mucocele of adjacent sinuses. Flow voids indicate a very vascular mass (e.g. a melanotic adenoma), whereas the more common carcinomas are less vascular. Both CT and MRI may demonstrate enlarged involved retropharyngeal lymph nodes (Ramos, Som and Solodnik, 1990).

Modern imaging techniques allow CT and MRI data to be viewed in similar projections, facilitating the choice of surgical approaches (Makielski, 1990).

Biopsy

Definitive diagnosis of malignancy depends on histopathology but the tumour cell type does not affect the treatment or prognosis of carcinomas. Amelanotic melanoma is particularly likely to be rapidly fatal (Berthelsen *et al.*, 1984). `

For a lesion within the antrum, access via a Caldwell–Luc-type approach is advisable to obtain an adequate specimen, and permits visualization of the neoplasm and palpation of the antral walls. However, now that CT scans can define the extent of the tumour, access via an intranasal antrostomy and using endoscopic instrumentation may be preferred in order to avoid removing the bone barrier between the tumour and the facial soft tissues. Biopsy of a lesion extending into the orbit or infratemporal region, or one invading the nose, is also best accomplished via an intranasal approach.

Tumours extending into the mouth can be biopsied easily. The specimen should be deep enough to provide tissue from the tumour and not just the thick, overlying palatal mucosa. When an ulcerated mass is present it is important to biopsy the adjacent non-ulcerated area, otherwise all that is demonstrated histologically may be non-specific necrotic tissue.

Classification and staging

A standardized classification of these relatively rare tumours is a prerequisite for recording the stage at which tumours present, comparing the results of different treatments and establishing the prognosis (Sakai, Shigematzu and Fuchihata, 1972; Harrison, 1978). Pooling of results from many centres enables the best treatment and advice to be given to individual patients.

Malignant tumours are traditionally classified by the TNM system: 'T' gives the size and extent of the primary tumour; 'N' indicates the state of the regional lymph nodes; and 'M' states whether or not distant metastases are present. The American Joint Committee on Cancer (AJCC) devised a staging system specifically for maxillary antrum tumours and modified it in 1988 (AJCC, 1988). The antrum is divided by an artificial 'plane of malignancy', running from the medial canthus of the eye to the angle of the mandible, into an anteroinferior 'infrastructure' and a posterosuperior 'suprastructure' (Ohngren, 1933). Malignancy in the suprastructure has usually involved bone at presentation.

Prognosis

Direction and extent of spread are probably the most important factors in prognosis and these in turn are related to tumour site and size at diagnosis. Zamora *et al.* (1990), in a retrospective study of 51 patients with localized primary malignancy of the maxillary sinus, found that the 5-year survival rate was 100% for T_1, 80% for T_2, 50% for T_3 and 5% for T_4. The probability of surviving 5 years after diagnosis was not related to the age at presentation, to the histological type of malignancy or to the treatment given, whether surgery alone, radiotherapy alone or surgery and radiotherapy in either order.

Tumour invasion of the orbital contents (T_4) carries a poorer prognosis than tumours with limited invasion of the orbital walls (T_3) (Zamora *et al.*, 1990). Superomedial extension may involve the ethmoid sinuses and thence the cranial base. Posterior extension carries the worst prognosis because the tumour reaches the base of the skull relatively quickly and clinical signs are absent until it is well advanced. Overall survival is low because diagnosis is often late. Melanotic melanoma is particularly likely to be rapidly fatal (Berthelsen *et al.*, 1984).

Treatment

Treatment, whether curative or palliative, is required because the natural history of antral malignancy is disfiguration followed by a slow, painful death from metastatic disease (Harrison, 1972).

Treatment options for carcinoma are surgery, radiotherapy or a combination of the two. Topical (Knegt *et al.*, 1985) and systemic chemotherapy (Siodlak *et al.*, 1990) have been added to the combination but the results have often been disappointing. Local intra-arterial infusion of cytotoxic drugs may be helpful for pain control, but this is more easily achieved with analgesics.

Melanomas require radical surgery, and radiotherapy is indicated only if the incision is incomplete, the tumour is inoperable or for recurrence (Berthelsen *et al.*, 1984).

In her comparison of surgical approaches to the skull base, Makielski (1990) states that, since the advent of CT and MRI, advances in intraoperative and postoperative monitoring and improvements in myocutaneous flaps have meant that surgery of the skull base has become more successful.

To obtain adequate posterior margins during removal of ethmomaxillary sinus carcinoma, extended maxillectomy with pterygomaxillary fossa dissection was designed by Fairbanks-Barbosa (1961). Tumour extending to the base of the skull through the infratemporal fossa may be removed using the mandibular swing to give good access (Biller, Shugar and Krespi, 1981), and a transfacial approach to the maxillary region is advocated by Hernandez Altemir (1986). Pterygoid *en bloc* dissection of recurrent tumour is a rapid radical procedure which provides good disease-free intervals in patients with a poor prognosis (Eilber and Zarem, 1977).

Surgery, whether it be intraoral (Figures 6.7 and 6.8) or a combined intraoral and extraoral operation, leaves a considerable defect, especially when removal of

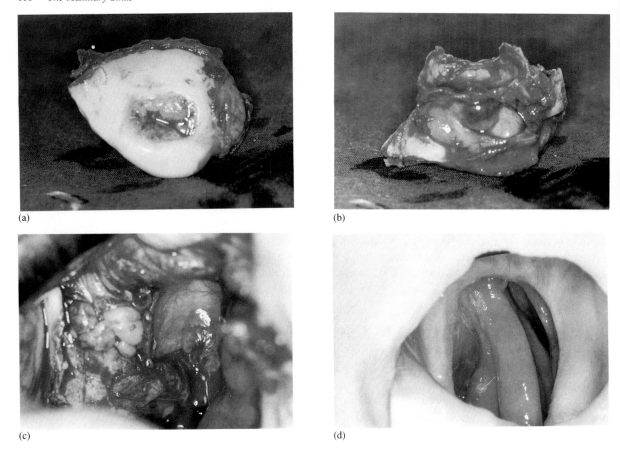

(a)

(b)

(c)

(d)

Figure 6.7 (a) and (b) Excision specimen and (c) tissue defect produced by removal of a palatal pleomorphic adenoma bulging into the sinus floor (b). The soft tissues were repaired and the residual defect (d) closed by an obturator

the eye and skin of the cheek is required (Figure 6.9). Reconstruction of the defect produced is a controversial topic. With the increasing use of microsurgical techniques, some surgeons advocate the transfer of myocutaneous flaps to fill the defect. This provides a one-stage reconstruction and a more acceptable result for the patient, though denture construction may be a problem. Critics of this technique claim that recurrence of tumour will be missed because it is covered up. Unfortunately, it is unlikely that such a recurrence would be operable anyway.

Langdon *et al.* (1991) grew oral keratinocytes in sheets from a lower labial mucosal biopsy and used this autologous keratinocyte graft to line the maxillectomy cavity after excision of a squamous cell carcinoma of the antrum. Epithelialization was complete in 3 weeks, and after 6 months the mucosa in the grafted area appeared healthy. This technique may avoid the candidal infection, hair growth and donor site pain which are problems with free split-skin lining grafts. Where there is an intraoral defect an obturator is fitted (Figures 6.8 and 6.9), which helps to fill out the cheek to some extent and improves facial appearance.

The Liverpool Head and Neck Oncology Group (1990) studied patients with end-stage squamous cell carcinoma of the head and neck, defined as advanced or

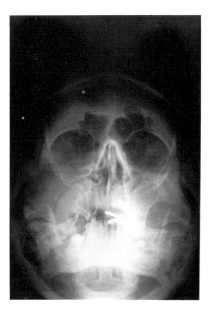

Figure 6.8 Occipitomental radiograph of a patient who had a right maxillectomy for carcinoma of the maxillary alveolus and sinus, and who has been wearing a large obturator for many years following the surgery, which proved curative. Part of the metallic structure of the obturator can be seen together with the clearly defined healed surgical defect

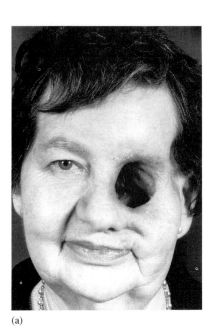

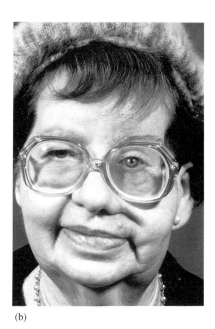

(a) (b)

Figure 6.9 (a) The healed surgical defect produced by left maxillectomy and extirpation of the orbit is obliterated by (b) an obturator and facial prosthesis attached to spectacles

recurrent disease no longer amenable to curative or palliative treatment with either surgery or radiotherapy. They found the median survival time was increased from 70 days in controls to 180 days in patients treated with cisplatin as a single chemotherapeutic agent. Combination with other chemotherapeutic agents (Liverpool Head and Neck Oncology Group, 1990) or alternation with other chemotherapeutic regimens (Siodlak *et al.*, 1990) does not increase survival time.

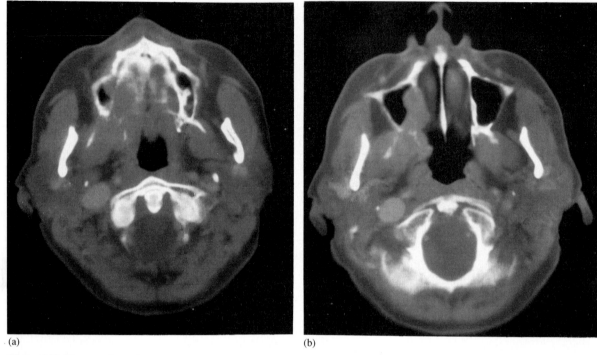

(a)   (b)

Figure 6.10 CT scans of a patient
with an adenoid cystic carcinoma
arising from the palatal minor
salivary glands and invading (a) the
palatal bone and (b) the sinus

Invasion of the maxillary sinus by local malignant disease

Tumours of the upper jaw spread easily into the sinus and are often impossible
to distinguish from those originating within it. Pleomorphic adenoma arising in
palatal minor salivary glands may bulge into the sinus floor (Figure 6.7a and b)
and adenoid cystic carcinoma may invade it (Figure 6.10).

Ramos, Som and Solodnik (1990) reported a case of nasopharyngeal
melanoma which invaded the maxillary sinus. The agressive nature of these
tumours is such that they have frequently invaded adjacent structures at
presentation (Barnes, 1985).

Metastatic carcinoma of the maxillary sinus

The maxillary sinus is a rare site for secondary tumour deposits. Kent and
Majumdar (1985) reviewed the literature since 1900 and found only 55 reported
cases of metastatic tumours of the maxillary sinus. The most common site of the
primary disease was the kidney (20 cases) followed by the breast in females and
the testicle (seminoma) in males. As adenocarcinoma in the antrum is so rare,
they suggest that any patient with a lesion of this histological type should have
an intravenous urogram (pyelogram) performed to exclude a renal primary. If
negative, it should be repeated during follow-up. Similarly, a bronchial primary
should be sought in a patient with an anaplastic tumour of the antrum.

References

AJCC (American Joint Committee on Cancer) (1988) *Malignant Disease of the Maxillary Sinus*, American Cancer Society, 90 Park Avenue, New York, NY 10016

Barnes, L. (ed.) (1985) *Surgical Pathology of the Head and Neck*, Vol. 1, 2nd edn, New York, Dekker, pp. 437–451

Barton, R. T. (1977) Nickel carcinogenesis of the respiratory tract. *Journal of Otolaryngology*, **6**, 412–422

Batsakis, J. G. (1979) *Tumors of the Head and Neck, Clinical and Pathological Considerations*, 2nd edn, Williams and Wilkins, Baltimore, chap. 7, pp. 177–187

Berthelsen, A., Anderson, A. P., Jensen, T. S. and Hansen, H. S. (1984) Melanomas of the mucosa in the oral cavity and the upper respiratory passages. *Cancer*, **54**, 907–912

Biller, H. F., Shugar, J. A. and Krespi, Y. P. (1981) A new technique for wide field exposure of the base of the skull. *Archives of Otolaryngology*, **105**, 99–107

Cheesman, A. D. (1987) Non-healing granulomata and tumours of the nose and sinuses. In *Scott-Brown's Otolaryngology*, Vol. 4, 5th edn (eds I. S. Mackay and T. R. Bull), Butterworth-Heinemann, Oxford, p. 300

Eilber, F. R. and Zarem, H. A. (1977) Pterygoid dissection for extensive cancer: an old concept revisited. *Plastic and Reconstructive Surgery*, **49**, 545–550

Fairbanks-Barbosa, J. (1961) Surgery of extensive cancer of the paranasal sinuses: presentation of a new technique. *Archives of Otolaryngology*, **73**, 129–138

Goren, A. D., Harley, N., Eisenbud, L., Levin, S. and Cohen, N. (1980) Clinical and radiobiologic features of Thorotrast-induced carcinoma of the maxillary sinus. A case report. *Oral Surgery*, **49**, 237–242

Harrison, D. F. N. (1971) The management of malignant tumors of nasal sinuses. *Otolaryngologic Clinics of North America*, **41**, 159–177

Harrison, D. F. N. (1972) The natural history of some cancers affecting the head and neck. *Journal of Laryngology and Otology*, **86**, 1189–1202

Harrison, D. F. N. (1978) Critical look at the classification of maxillary sinus carcinomata. *Annals of Otolaryngology*, **87**, 3–9

Hernandez Altemir, F. (1986) Transfacial access to the retromaxillary area. *Journal of Maxillofacial Surgery*, **14**, 165–170

Higginson, J. and Oettle, A. G. (1960) Cancer incidence in the Bantu and 'Cape Colored' races of South Africa: report of a cancer survey in the Transvaal (1953–55). *Journal of the National Cancer Institute*, **24**, 589–671

Hole, D. (1991) Personal communication

Kent, S. E. and Majumdar, B. (1985) Metastatic tumours in the maxillary sinus. A report of two cases and a review of the literature. *Journal of Laryngology and Otology*, **99**, 459–462

Knegt, P. P., De Jong, P. C., Van Andel, J. G., De Boer, M. F., Eykenboom, W. and Van Der Schans, E. (1985) Carcinoma of the paranasal sinuses. *Cancer*, **56**, 57–62

Langdon, J., Williams, D. M., Navsaria, H. and Leigh, I. M. (1991) Autologous keratinocyte grafting: a new technique for intra-oral reconstruction. *British Dental Journal*, **171**, 87–90

The Liverpool Head and Neck Oncology Group (1990) A phase III randomised trial of cisplatinum, methotrexate, cisplatinum + methotrexate, and cisplatinum + 5-FU in end stage squamous carcinoma of the head and neck. *British Journal of Cancer*, **61**, 311–315

McGregor, I. A. and McGregor, F. M. (1986) *Cancer of the Face and Mouth: Pathology and Management for Surgeons*, Churchill Livingstone, Edinburgh

Makielski, K. H. (1990) Comparison of surgical approaches to the skull base. *Journal of Otolaryngology*, **19**, 242–248

Mundy, E. A., Neiders, M. E., Sako, K. and Greene, G. W. (1985) Maxillary sinus cancer: a study of 33 cases. *Journal of Oral Pathology*, **14**, 27–36

Ohngren, L. G. (1933) Malignant tumours of the maxillo-ethmoidal region. *Acta Oto-laryngologica. Supplement (Stockholm)*, **18–20**, 103–105

Ramos, R., Som, P. M. and Solodnik, P. (1990) Case Report. Nasopharyngeal melanotic melanoma: MRI characteristics. *Journal of Computer Assisted Tomography*, **14**, 997–999

Sakai, S., Shigematzu, Y. and Fuchihata, H. (1972) Diagnosis and TNM classification of maxillary sinus carcinoma. *Acta Oto-laryngologica, (Stockholm)* **74**, 123–129

Sakai, S., Murata, M., Sasaki, R., Tsujimoto, T., Miyaguchi, M. and Hohki, A. (1983) Combined therapy for maxillary sinus carcinoma with special reference to cryosurgery. *Rhinology*, **21**, 179–184

Siodlak, M. Z., Stell, P. M., Wilson, J. A. *et al.* (1990) Alternating cisplatinum and VAC ineffective in end stage squamous cell carcinoma of the head and neck. *Journal of Laryngology and Otology,* **104,** 631–633

Zamora, R. L., Harvey, J. E., Sessions, D. G., Spector, J. G. and Spitznagel, E. L. Jr (1990) Clinical classification and staging for primary malignancies of the maxillary antrum. *Laryngoscope,* **100,** 1106–1111

Chapter 7

Cysts involving the maxillary sinus

Cysts are abnormal fluid-filled cavities usually lined by epithelium. They are most frequent in the tooth-bearing parts of the jaws, apparently due to the many epithelial cell rests remaining after odontogenesis. A great variety of cysts can be found in the maxillary sinus, arising either from the maxillary alveolus and encroaching on the sinus, or directly from the lining of the sinus itself. The distinction is of practical importance since associated dental disease may require treatment for its own sake or to eliminate an underlying cause.

Cysts can be asymptomatic and so reach a considerable size before diagnosis. They come to attention either because of the effects of growth of a space-occupying lesion or as incidental findings on radiographic examination. Occasionally they become infected and lead to acute symptoms (see Figure 4.4). Initial diagnosis is by further radiographic examination, using either plain radiography or more sophisticated tomography, or by removal and histopathological examination. In view of the special features of lesions of this area, and especially the rich variety of odontogenic lesions, the opinion of an oral pathologist is invaluable.

Non-odontogenic cysts

Mucosal antral cysts

The mucosal antral cysts are the most common lesions affecting the maxillary antrum. The variety of names given to these lesions reflects the obscurity of their pathogenesis. Paperella (1963) avoided the controversy and simply called them 'mucosal antral cysts'. Killey and Kay (1970) added the term 'benign' to indicate their innocuous nature. The reported incidence in radiographic surveys varies from 2% to 10% of the population studied. The type of radiograph used varies from series to series but there does seem to be a variation between different populations. Most of these cysts arise from the antral floor and so may be seen on an orthopantomogram as well as on a Waters' projection (Figure 7.1). The increasing number of such radiographs being taken may lead to an increased frequency of observation of these usually asymptomatic lesions. Two types have been described, secretory and non-secretory, the latter being more common. Allard, Van der Kwast and Van der Waal (1981) reviewed the literature and the possible causes.

The secretory type, or mucous retention cyst, probably arises from obstruction of a gland outlet during a period of altered secretion in response to sinus infection or allergy. Continued secretion causes dilatation of the gland, resulting in a cyst lined with epithelium.

Figure 7.1 Mucous cyst of the right maxillary sinus

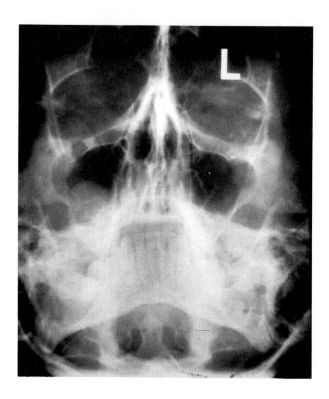

The non-secreting type, or mucous extravasation cyst, occurs when fluid accumulates in the subepithelial tissues. Capillary damage permits protein leakage into the sinus mucosa which has become oedematous due to infection or allergy. The cyst formed in this way has an inner lining of flattened fibroblasts and contains an ultrafiltrate of blood serum. It is therefore similar to the oral mucosal mucous extravasation cyst or mucocele.

Signs and Symptoms

These cysts are usually asymptomatic and are found by chance on radiography. Cases have been reported (Bret-Day, 1960) where symptomless buccal expansion was the presenting sign, and Shear (1983) describes a case with an intraoral fluctuant swelling, but these are unusual presentations. Spontaneous discharge or prolapse into the nose is common and therefore bone expansion is rare.

Paperella (1963) found that large cysts produced symptoms of headache, usually described as a heavy feeling in the orbital or frontal region on the affected side, whereas small cysts only occasionally gave symptoms.

Symptoms may be caused by fluid within large cysts compressing the underlying antral mucosa, by blockage of the ostium compromising aeration of the sinus, or, as Stammberger and Wolf (1988) suggest, by activation of local reflexes by mucosal contact and release of neuropeptides such as substance P.

Radiology

Antral cysts are usually seen as dome-shaped radiopacities arising from the floor or lateral wall of the sinus (Figure 7.1). They have a broad base and usually occur singly alongside adjacent mucosa of normal appearance. Antral polyps with an allergic or infective aetiology may also project from any of the walls but tend to be multiple and are associated with generalized thickening of the antral mucosa.

Normal sinus wall structures such as vascular channels are still visible superimposed on the opacity of mucosal antral cysts, and unlike odontogenic cysts they lack the radiopaque outline which indicates a bony margin. Being rounded, the mucosal antral cyst does not fill the inner and upper angles of the antrum, producing a characteristic small dark triangle on radiographs (Killey and Kay, 1970). The angle between the floor of the sinus and the antral cyst is also said to be more acute than that produced by a cyst 'expanding' into the sinus. There is a site predilection for the angle between the facial wall and the medial wall in the floor of the sinus which might be explained by turgid, swollen lining lifting off the underlying sharply-curved bone surface.

Treatment

Benign antral cysts vary in size and seem to be slow growing. Gothberg *et al.* (1976) followed up a series of mucosal cysts over a 10-year period and observed no significant increase in size. Asymptomatic maxillary mucosal antral cysts do not require treatment.

Symptomatic cysts may be decompressed by antral puncture or intranasal antrostomy, or removed via the canine fossa approach. The cysts have a very thin bluish wall and tend to puncture and collapse on removal. The collapsed cyst can be separated from the surrounding antral mucosa by simple traction. Fisher, Whittet and Croft (1989) deflated painful mucosal antral cysts via the sublabial route by aspirating them under endoscopic control. The ostium and the remaining sinus mucosa could then be conveniently inspected.

Surgical maxillary cyst

The surgical maxillary or postoperative cyst develops in epithelium trapped in the wound at operation for sinusitis. It was first described, as a surgical ciliated cyst, by Gregory and Shafer (1958). It has a higher incidence in Japan where maxillary sinus surgery is frequent. Patients who have had surgery to the maxillary sinus 10–30 years previously present with buccal swelling with pain and purulent discharge.

Radiographically a well-defined radiolucency is seen but, apart from the lack of association of a tooth, there are no distinctive features to differentiate it from a cyst of dental origin.

Treatment is by enucleation. The cyst consists of a thin fibrous tissue wall lined by epithelium which is usually ciliated. There may be areas of cubical or squamous epithelium and occasionally there is no epithelium at all.

Cyst of controversial origin

Globulomaxillary cyst

According to Smith (1968), globulomaxillary cysts have a tendency to involve the maxillary sinus or extend to the roof of the mouth, or both. They are usually asymptomatic and are an incidental radiographic discovery. They appear as a well-defined radiolucency, shaped like an inverted pear, between the roots of the upper lateral incisor and canine. The roots of these teeth are divergent and the teeth are vital to pulp testing.

It was thought that in embryonic life discrete facial processes covered in epithelium came together and fused and fissural cysts arose from remnants of the epithelium which failed to disintegrate. It is now known that there are centres of growth covered by a continuous sheet of epithelium and demarcated by furrows. Defective growth of mesenchyme in the region of the facial furrow might still result in enclavement of epithelium. Christ (1970) reviewed the literature and concluded that cysts of this type are odontogenic, and Wysocki (1981) reviewed 37 cases presenting as 'globulomaxillary cysts' in this way which he found to be various odontogenic and other lesions. Little and Jakobsen (1988) consider the evidence inconclusive and neither the odontogenic nor the fissural hypothesis disproved. 'Globulomaxillary' is perhaps best considered as a clinical term which simply denotes the position of a cyst. The cyst is enucleated and submitted for histological examination. The diagnosis will determine the further management of the patient.

Odontogenic cysts

All odontogenic cysts arise from odontogenic epithelium but at different stages of tooth development. (Seward, Harris and McGowan, 1987)

Periapical cysts

These inflammatory odontogenic cysts are the most common of all cysts of the oral region (Lucas, 1984). They occur most frequently between the ages of 20 and 60 years, with a male to female ratio of 3:2. They are found three times more often in the maxilla than in the mandible. An apical cyst from an upper canine, premolar or molar, and occasionally even a lateral incisor, may enlarge sufficiently to encroach on the maxillary sinus (Figure 7.2). They are believed to arise when epithelial rests of Malassez are stimulated to grow by chronic inflammation. There is a history of caries, infection or trauma to the involved tooth. If uninfected, they may remain asymptomatic and may be found incidentally on radiographs. The associated tooth will be non-vital and may be discoloured.

When the cyst enlarges into the maxillary sinus it can reach a considerable size before causing symptoms (Figure 7.3). As growth of the cyst continues, the sinus floor becomes gradually thinned and the cyst bulges into the lumen and eventually contacts and adheres to the mucoperiosteal lining. The whole sinus cavity can become occupied by the cyst, and occasionally there may be expansion and even erosion of its walls (Figure 7.3).

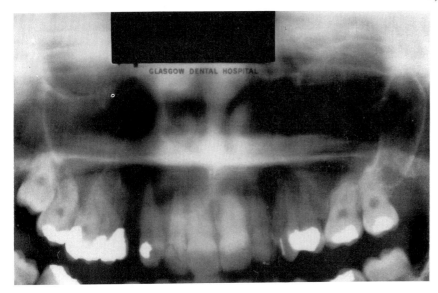

Figure 7.2 Periapical cyst arising from the upper right canine tooth which is bulging into the right maxillary sinus but is separated from it by a bony margin

Radiology

The tooth from which an apical cyst has arisen lacks an intact lamina dura at its apex. The cysts appear initially as a radiolucency within bone but when they enlarge into the antrum apical cysts are seen as relatively radiopaque because the fluid within the cyst is more dense than the air which normally fills the sinus. They are oval or circular in outline with a well-defined radiopaque margin indicating a surrounding lamina of bone. This bone lacks vascular channels, which are a normal structural feature of the sinus wall. Periapical and anterior or oblique occlusal radiographs are useful for demonstrating these details.

Residual cysts

Residual cysts are cysts which remain after the associated tooth is exfoliated or extracted or a periapical cyst is incompletely removed. They are therefore more common in older patients, but are also more common in the maxilla than the mandible. An edentulous patient may complain of increasing tightness of the upper denture or, conversely, of looseness from underlying swelling and displacement. The denture may have been relieved in order to accommodate an increasing buccal swelling. In the case of a large lesion there may even be swelling of the cheek.

Treatment

Enucleation of the cyst and root filling or extraction of the involved teeth will usually produce bone regeneration and healing. Marsupialization of apical cysts in the maxilla is unsatisfactory as the residual defect usually persists, and this

Figure 7.3 (a) Lipiodol has been injected into an extensive cyst in the right maxilla which has occupied most of the sinus. (b) The cyst arises from the upper lateral incisor and, unusually, crosses the midline

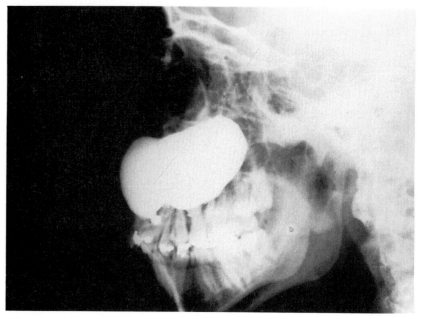

(a)

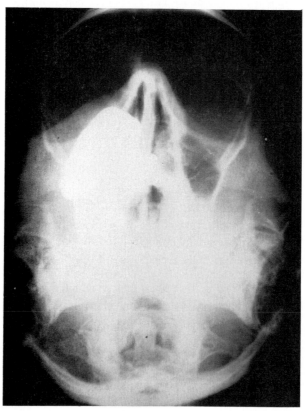

(b)

is especially so in the anterior region. At operation every effort should be made to strip the cyst lining completely from the bony cavity. This is an easy task unless there has been recent decompression and consequent shrinkage, such as can occur after diagnostic aspiration, or infection and discharge or drainage. In these circumstances, separation of cyst lining from newly formed rough-surfaced bone is more difficult than from smoother, mature compact bone. Separation of cyst lining from sinus lining when they are back to back with no intervening bone is more difficult, but it is always worth attempting. Healing is usually uneventful and the antrum reverts to its size prior to the presence of the cyst.

Dentigerous cyst

The most common form arises by enlargement of the follicular space about the whole or part of the crown of a tooth. The enamel organ becomes cystic after amelogenesis is complete. Fluid accumulates between the crown and the reduced enamel epithelium or within the reduced enamel epithelium (Seward, Harris and McGowan, 1987).

The dentigerous cyst is the next most common odontogenic lesion after the apical cyst. Dentigerous cysts can be divided histologically into follicular dentigerous cysts, which are lined by cells derived from the reduced enamel epithelium, and extrafollicular dentigerous cysts, which arise from the dental lamina and produce keratin.

The teeth most commonly involved in cyst formation are the mandibular third molar, followed by the maxillary canine: that is, teeth which erupt late. The sex incidence is equal and diagnosis is usually made during childhood and adolescence. Cystic expansion is rapid and an upper third molar may be displaced up the posterolateral wall (Figure 7.4) and an upper canine up the facial wall of the maxillary sinus to its roof. Expansion of the anterior maxilla by a cyst involving the upper canine often occurs and may be mistaken for acute sinusitis or cellulitis. The tooth may also be displaced medially (Chuong, 1984). However, it is usually the facial or posterolateral wall of the sinus which is eroded. Often the cyst is extensive at diagnosis, and a case of a dentigerous cyst arising from a supernumerary incisor and involving both sinuses was reported by Most and Roy (1982).

The lesions are often asymptomatic and a well-defined unilocular radiolucency associated with the crown of an unerupted tooth is noticed incidentally on a radiograph which perhaps may be taken to help account for the associated tooth missing from the arch. When the cyst is first palpable it is as a hard bony swelling in the buccal sulcus, but as it enlarges further the overlying bone becomes thinner until it feels like pieces of egg shell, and later the swelling becomes fluctuant and has a blue hue. An aggressive dentigerous cyst may produce bony expansion sufficient to cause facial asymmetry, extreme tooth displacement, root resorption and pain.

Treatment is usually by enucleation, although marsupialization may be performed if the tooth is to be retained in the hope of eruption, which, however, is less likely than in the case of a mandibular lesion. The cyst usually has a thick lining containing yellow fluid and cholesterol crystals which shimmer when they are put on to a dry swab and viewed in a bright light.

Figure 7.4 A large dentigerous cyst including the upper right third molar and occupying the right maxillary sinus. (a) The first orthopantomogram was taken to locate the missing third molar which is only just visible at the extreme top edge of the radiograph and is partially obscured by the label. (b) Part of a second radiograph taken at a higher level shows the tooth and the associated cyst very clearly. The (c) occipitomental, and (d) and (e) true lateral films demonstrate the high medial position of the tooth. The difference in clarity of the image of the tooth between the left and right lateral views shows the advantage in favour of the film positioned on the affected side and therefore closer to its object

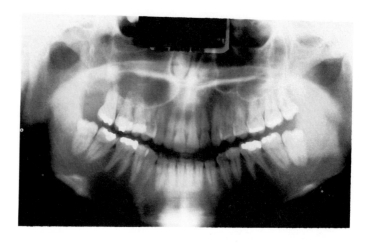

(a)

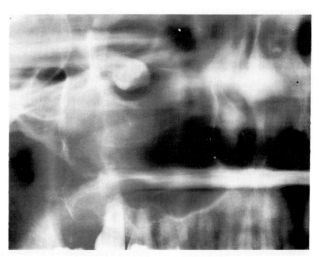

(b)

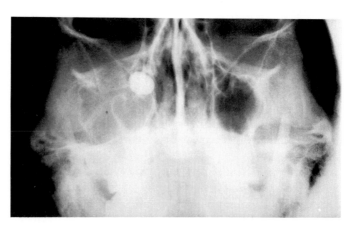

(c)

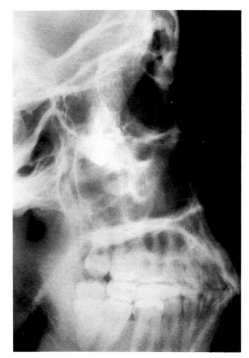

(d)

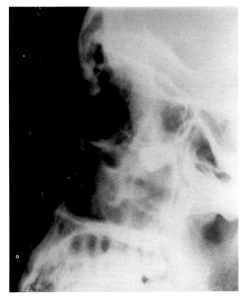

(e)

Odontogenic keratocyst

The diagnosis of odontogenic keratocyst is histological. There are no pathogno-monic clinical features but bony expansion is common. All primordial cysts and those of the basal cell naevus–bifid rib syndrome (Gorlin–Goltz syndrome) are odontogenic keratocysts. Dentigerous cysts and occasionally apical periodontal cysts may be keratocysts. The odontogenic keratocysts in the Gorlin–Goltz syndrome are often multiple. Although they usually develop at an early age, when they may deform and displace developing teeth, their presence may not become apparent until middle age. As with all keratocysts, the recurrence rate is high. Because ameloblastomas may develop in the cysts of this syndrome, thorough surgical removal and histological examination are essential. Patients with arachnodactyly may have multiple odontogenic cysts of the maxilla and mandible (Oatis,Burch and Samuels, 1971).

Recognition of this type of cyst is important because of its high recurrence rate. The odontogenic keratocyst has many features in common with the ameloblastoma, including the mean age at diagnosis, a predilection for the mandible (with only 20% occurring in the maxilla), its radiographic appearance and its tendency to recur after surgical removal.

Radiology

Radiographically the odontogenic keratocyst has a thin sclerotic border produced by reactive bone formation. It may be smooth or scalloped and the lesion may be unilocular or multilocular. These cysts often appear to be dentigerous cysts and sometimes cause resorption of the roots of nearby teeth.

Histology

The cyst wall, which often shows infolding, is composed of stratified squamous epithelium, only six to eight cells thick and lacking rete pegs. The cyst cavity contains masses of keratin and less soluble protein than the patient's serum. There is a very limited thickness of surrounding fibrous capsule and the cyst wall is fragile and friable; as it is so easily torn during removal, the retention of fragments may be a factor in recurrence. Epithelial dysplasia occurs in the lining, and the connective tissue of the wall often shows islands of epithelium or satellite cysts which may also contribute to the tendency to recur. Carcinomatous change has been reported but, though apparently more frequent in keratocysts than non-keratinizing dental cysts, it is fortunately very rare.

Treatment

Treatment is surgical by marsupialization or enucleation. Years of postoperative review are necessary because of the high recurrence rate.

Calcifying epithelial odontogenic cyst (Pindborg tumour)

Thirty per cent of these cysts occur in the maxilla. Radiographically they usually appear as a well-defined radiolucency containing variable amounts of calcification. The epithelial lining consists of columnar or cuboidal cells and the cyst contains large numbers of ghost epithelial cells which have keratinized or calcified. They may grow very large and involve the maxillary sinus but do not recur after complete excision.

Differential diagnosis

Radiology

All cystic lesions involving the maxillary sinuses need to be localized by extraoral radiographs taken at right angles to each other. Occasionally CT scans may be necessary to determine whether erosion of the medial wall of the sinus has occurred.

Cysts arising from the anterior teeth and involving the maxillary sinus are usually larger in the anteroposterior dimension than those arising from the posterior teeth.

There may be difficulty in distinguishing a cyst in the antrum from a locule of the sinus itself. Vascular channels are seen in the wall of the normal sinus (see Figure 3.5) but not in the expanded bone covering a cyst. Symmetry, seen particularly on occlusal films, is indicative of normality because symmetrical pathology, though possible, is highly unlikely. If doubt cannot be resolved then recourse to aspiration may be justified, though perhaps not in the absence of symptoms.

Antroscopy

Direct inspection of the maxillary sinus with an endoscope (see Chapter 3) gives a more accurate diagnosis of mucosal antral cysts than radiology, and treatment may be carried out at the same time.

Aspiration

Ameloblastomas and other solid odontogenic tumours may have a dentigerous relationship to an unerupted tooth and it may be difficult, particularly in the edentulous patient, to determine whether a radiolucency is the maxillary antrum or a cyst. Aspiration via the buccal approach intraorally will provide useful information.

The area is anaesthetized, a hole is drilled through mucosa and bone plate with a small bur, and a wide-bore needle on a syringe is inserted. If air only is aspirated the maxillary sinus has been entered. Failure to withdraw the plunger of the syringe suggests that the lesion is solid, and aspiration of fluid indicates a cyst or infected antrum. Straw-coloured fluid, in which yellow cholesterol crystals are seen when the fluid is smeared on to gauze, indicates an apical, residual or dentigerous cyst, and mucus indicates a benign mucous cyst. Pus is present when there is an infected cyst or sinus and should be submitted for microscopy, culture and sensitivity testing. Aspiration of an odontogenic keratocyst yields a thick yellow inspissated material, resembling pus but without the odour.

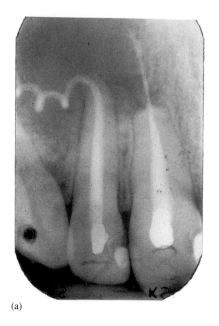

(a)

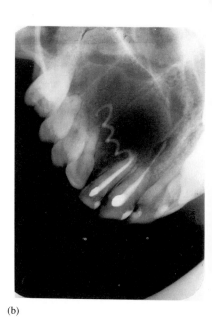

(b)

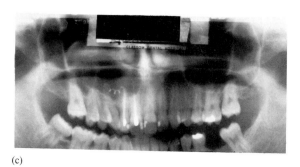

(c)

Figure 7.5 A 20-year-old drama student noticed fullness of his right cheek and altered vocal resonance on the right side. (a) Periapical and (b) occlusal radiographs revealed a large cyst in the right maxilla and its origin from the root-filled lateral incisor. (c) An orthopantomogram, and (d) occipitomental views demonstrated the size and extent of the cyst. The cyst was enucleated and postoperative films (e, f, g, h, i), show satisfactory healing and eventual restoration of sinus symmetry

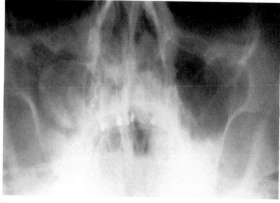

(d)

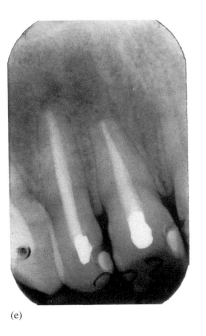

(e)

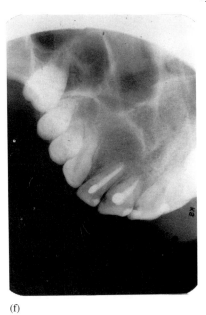

(f)

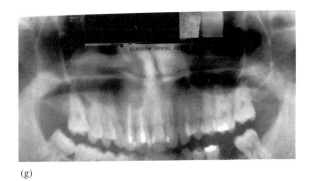

(g)

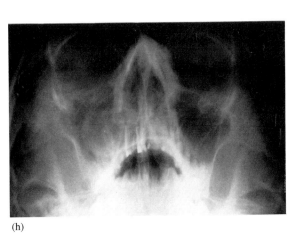

(h)

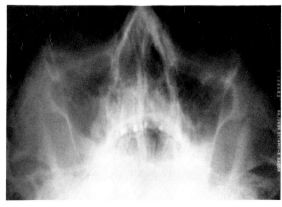

(i)

Treatment

An incision along the buccal gingival margin from, if necessary, the upper third molar region to the midline permits the raising of a mucoperiosteal flap (Figure 7.6a). An anterior relieving incision into the depth of the sulcus may facilitate retraction of the flap if the cyst has caused a pronounced buccal swelling. If the cyst is fluctuant, extra care must be taken to avoid tearing the lining during its separation from the overlying mucoperiosteum. The flap is reflected by undermining the mucoperiosteum with a broad-bladed periosteal elevator, working on the surface of sound bone well clear of lesion on either side (Figure 7.6b). The infraorbital nerve should be identified and avoided by careful placement of retractors. The bony defect should be approached from each direction in turn, working along the bone surface and turning back the periosteum until the margin of the defect is reached. The defect is enlarged, or if none is present bone is removed, to give access to the cyst, taking care not to damage the apices of adjacent teeth (Figure 7.6c). The plane between the cyst lining and the

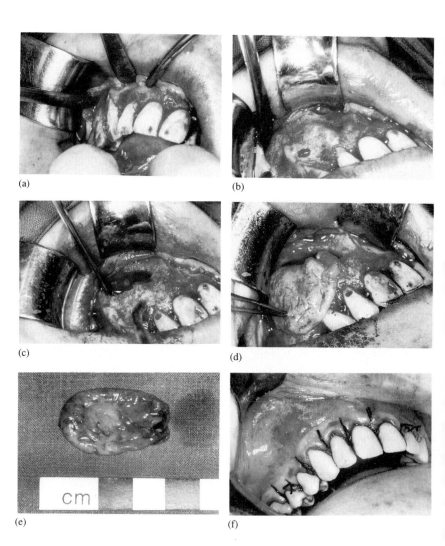

(a)   (b)

(c)   (d)

(e)   (f)

Figure 7.6 Removal of the cyst shown radiographically in Figure 7.5. The stages of the operation are described in the text. A flap is raised (a), and the bone surface widely exposed (b). Bone overlying the cyst is removed (c). The cyst is enucleated from its cavity and removed (d), and the apical seal of the incisors is checked. The cyst lining is dispatched for histological examination, (e). The flap is sutured back in position (f) and healed without problems.

bony cavity is identified and the cyst lining is easily stripped from its overlying bone or, with more difficulty, gently separated from underlying sinus mucosa. Complete removal of the cyst lining is especially difficult inferiorly, where the roots of the teeth produce a complex shape to the sinus floor, but can usually be accomplished with careful dissection (Figure 7.6d). Because cysts are usually lined by squamous epithelium which lacks the cilia required to beat secretions toward the ostium, retention of the inferior cyst wall would hinder mucociliary clearance of the sinus. The ideal result in a moderate-sized cyst is complete removal of the cyst lining while leaving the sinus mucosa intact. This size of defect can be allowed to fill with blood clot and will be obliterated by replacement with granulation tissue, scar and new bone formation (Figure 7.5e-i). In the case of larger lesions the remaining sinus cavity is sought and opened widely, so converting the defect into an extension of the sinus. It can be packed with ribbon gauze soaked in Whitehead's varnish and externalized via a temporary inferior meatal antrostomy, or a tube drain can be passed by the same route. If normal sinus function was present before operation, these procedures are unnecessary. Closure is with 3/0 silk sutures (Figure 7.6f) and the patient is given antibiotics, nasal drops and inhalations, as in the regimen detailed in Chapter 4.

Removal of a pack or drain can be accomplished by anaesthetizing the nostril with ribbon gauze soaked in 3 ml cocaine 10% for 5–10 minutes and providing sedation if required. Sutures are removed 10–14 days after surgery. Postoperative review of the vitality of associated teeth and radiographic monitoring of bone deposition is advised. Non-vital teeth should be root filled and if extraction becomes necessary it should be delayed until healing is as far advanced as possible. All cysts involving the maxillary antrum should be examined histopathologically to confirm the clinical diagnosis and exclude the possibility of malignant change.

Seward and Seward (1968) reviewed the techniques available for the treatment of cysts of the maxilla and described their development.

References

Allard, R. H. B., Van der kwast, W. A. M. and Van der waal, I. (1981) Mucosal antral cysts. *Oral Surgery, Oral Medicine, Oral Pathology*, **51**, 1–9

Bret-Day, R. C. (1960) Secretory cyst of the maxillary antrum presenting with oral symptoms. *British Dental Journal*, **109**, 268–270

Christ, T. F. (1970) The globulomaxillary cyst: an embryologic misconception. *Oral Surgery*, **30**, 515–526

Chuong, R. (1984) Dentigerous cysts involving maxillary sinus. *Journal of the American Dental Association*, **109**, 59–60

Fisher, E. W., Whittet, H. B. and Croft, C. B. (1989) Symptomatic mucosal cysts of the maxillary sinus: antroscopic treatment. *Journal of Laryngology and Otology*, **103**, 1184–1186

Gothberg, K. A., Little, J. W., King, D. R. and Bean, L. R. (1976) A clinical study of cysts arising from the mucosa of the maxillary sinus. *Oral Surgery, Oral Medicine, Oral Pathology*, **41**, 52–58

Gregory, G. T. and Shafer, W. G. (1958) Surgical ciliated cysts of the maxilla: report of cases. *Journal of Oral Surgery*, **16**, 251–253

Killey, H. C. and Kay, L. W. (1970) Benign mucosal cysts of the maxillary sinus. *International Surgery*, **53**, 235–244

Little, J. W. and Jakobsen, J. O. (1988) Origin of the globulomaxillary cyst *Journal of Oral Surgery*, **31**, 188–195

Lucas, R. B. (1984) *Pathology of Tumours of Oral Tissues*, 4th edn, Churchill Livingstone, Edinburgh

Most, D. S. and Roy, E. P. (1982) A large dentigerous cyst associated with a supernumerary tooth. *Journal of Oral and Maxillofacial Surgery*, **40,** 119–120

Oatis, G. W. Jr, Burch, M. S. and Samuels, H. S. (1971) Marfan's syndrome with multiple mandibular and maxillary cysts: report of a case. *Journal of Oral Surgery*, **29,** 515–519

Paperella, M. M. (1963) Mucosal cysts of the maxillary sinus. *Archives of Otolaryngology*, **77,** 650–657

Seward, G. R., Harris, M. and McGowan D. A. (1987) Cysts of the jaws. Killey and Kay's *Outline of Oral Surgery*, Part I, Wright, Bristol, pp. 263–296

Seward, M. H. and Seward, G. R. (1968) Observations on Snawdon's technique for the treatment of cysts in the maxilla. *British Journal of Oral Surgery*, **6,** 149–160

Shear, M. (1983) Cysts associated with the maxillary antrum. In *Cysts of the Oral Regions*, 2nd edn, Wright, Bristol, pp. 160–165

Smith, H. W. (1968) Cystic lesions of the maxilla. I. Classification and clinical Features. *Archives of Otolaryngology*, **88,** 113–123

Stammberger, H. and Wolf, G. (1988) Headaches and sinus disease: the endoscopic approach. *Annals of Otology, Rhinology and Laryngology*, **97,** (Suppl. 134)

Wysocki, G. P. (1981) The differential diagnosis of globulomaxillary radiolucencies. *Oral Surgery, Oral Medicine, Oral Pathology*, **51,** 281–286

Chapter 8

Other diseases involving the maxillary sinus

Certain diseases do not primarily affect the maxillary sinus but may involve it by invasion or expansion into it (Shafer, Hine and Levy, 1983); some of these are discussed below.

Developmental abnormalities

Crouzon syndrome

Early synostosis of the sutures produces hypoplasia of the maxillae, and therefore the maxillary sinuses, together with a high arched palate.

Treacher Collins syndrome

Mandibulofacial dysostosis is associated with grossly and symmetrically underdeveloped maxillary sinuses and malar bones.

Binder syndrome

Maxillonasal dysplasia (the Binder syndrome) involves hypoplasia of the middle third of the face. There is maxillary retrognathism, smaller maxillary length and frontal and maxillary sinus hypoplasia. This syndrome may be associated with cleft palate, suggesting either a field effect of a teratogen on the developing mid-face or a genetic aetiology (Mossey and Sandham, 1989).

Haemangioma

Sheppard and Mickelson (1990) report a haemangioma affecting the maxillary sinus, and Darlow *et al.* (1988) an extensive anteriovenous malformation.

Diseases in bone

Fibrous dysplasia

Fibrous dysplasia is a disease of bone that can affect one site (monostotic) or several bones (polyostotic). If it is associated with cutaneous pigmentation, endocrine dysfunction and precocious puberty, the polyostotic form is known as the Albright syndrome. Monostotic fibrous dysplasia, although less severe than the polyostotic form, is of more interest to dental surgeons because of the frequency with which the jaws are affected. Despite the similarity of the two forms of fibrous dysplasia, the monostotic form has not been observed to progress to the polyostotic form.

The aetiology of monostotic fibrous dysplasia is unknown. It presents more commonly in children and young adults than in older persons. The maxilla is affected more often than the mandible and usually the earliest clinical sign is a localized swelling. The swelling is painless and commonly involves the labial or buccal plate, while the overlying mucosa is normal in appearance. When the maxilla is involved the maxillary sinus can be almost completely obliterated, but this does not lead to any sinus symptoms (Figure 8.1). The floor of the orbit and base of skull may also become affected. The lesion is not encapsulated, and increasing facial deformity occurs as a result of local spread and growths. Intraorally, there may be some tipping or spacing of the teeth as the lesion expands, together with tenderness of the swollen area, which can lead to confusion with an inflammatory lesion (Figure 8.2).

Radiological features

The radiographic appearance varies, depending on the amount of osseous tissue present, from a distinct well-circumscribed small unilocular radiolucency, through a rather larger multilocular radiolucency, to a more dense and diffuse ground-glass appearance (Figure 8.1). Where the ground-glass appearance is seen, the lesion is not well demarcated and blends into the surrounding bone. The roots of the involved teeth may be separated but resorption is rare.

Histopathology

Considerable variation is seen microscopically, but the lesion is essentially a mass of fibrous tissue containing irregular islands of trabeculae of immature woven (alamellar) bone. The cellularity of the fibrous stroma varies a great deal.

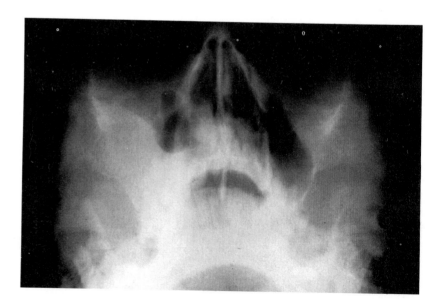

Figure 8.1 Occipitomental radiograph of an 18-year-old girl with fibrous dysplasia affecting the right maxilla

Treatment

Definitive surgical treatment to correct the facial deformity should be delayed until skeletal growth ceases because progression of monostotic fibrous dysplasia slows or is arrested at this time. However, concern about the deteriorating facial appearance often dictates conservative removal of a portion of the lesion causing the deformity at an earlier stage, via an intraoral approach. A gingival margin incision is made and a mucoperiosteal flap raised. The cut surface is trimmed using a combination of chisels, bone rongeurs and a handpiece with large burs. The bone may bleed profusely and haemostasis should be obtained before closure to avoid haematoma and the possibility of new bone formation. Patients should be warned that the deformity will recur and that further surgery may then be necessary. In the more aggressive form of the disease, where extension to the base of the skull and orbit make conservative treatment less acceptable, block resection of the actively diseased bone, with reconstruction by means of split cranial grafts, has been suggested to eliminate the disease and prevent the development of a virtually untreatable facial deformity.

Although fibrous dysplasia is considered to be a benign disease, cases of spontaneous malignant transformation into sarcoma, usually osteosarcoma, have been reported (Schwartz and Alpert, 1964). Cases of sarcoma developing in patients who had previously had their fibrous dysplasia treated by irradiation have also been recorded (Tanner, Dahlin and Childs, 1961).

Ossifying fibroma

This condition can occur in the maxilla and encroach on the sinus. It is a form of fibro-osseous lesion which tends to be well demarcated from surrounding normal bone and it has a variable tendency for growth. Some cases are aggressive, while others reach a steady state and become densely calcified. The actively growing type has to be distinguished from osteosarcoma, and though the radiographic appearance alone may be differentiated from the classical radiating

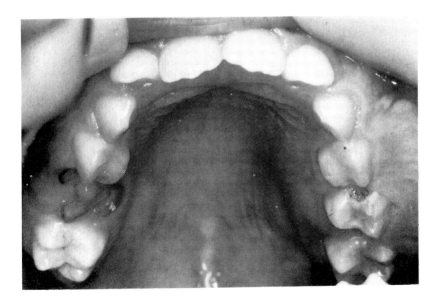

Figure 8.2 Fibrous dysplasia of the left maxilla in a young boy. The carious left second deciduous molar was originally assumed to be the source of the swelling but the signs of acute infection are absent

pattern, biopsy is essential to establish the diagnosis. The opinion of a pathologist with specialist knowledge of bone and jaw lesions is essential because the histological appearance of the whole range of fibro-osseous and giant cell lesions is highly variable and interpretation is difficult.

Giant cell lesions

The heterogeneous nature of lesions containing a predominance of giant cells continues to engender debate. The maxilla is a very rare site of such lesions and reports of maxillary sinus invasion are sparse. Smith, Marrogi and Delfino (1990) report a case of multifocal giant cell lesions in which lesions were found simultaneously in both sinuses some years after resection of a similar lesion in the mandible. In any case of giant cell lesion of the jaws, the possibility of hyperparathyroidism as a primary cause must be ruled out by biochemical estimations of serum calcium, phosphate, alkaline phosphatase and hormone levels. Harris (1990) states that calcitonin cures central giant cell granulomas of the jaws and therefore their surgical removal is no longer indicated.

Paget's disease

Paget's disease or osteitis deformans was first described by Sir James Paget in 1877. Its aetiology is unknown but it has been suggested recently that slow virus infections with a parvovirus carried by pet dogs may explain the patchy prevalence. Otherwise there must be a genetic predisposition as it is exceedingly rare in racial groups other than North Europeans and their descendants, irrespective of their place of residence. It chiefly affects patients over 40 years of age but may start in the teens (McGowan, 1974). Symptoms develop slowly and the disease follows a chronic course. The main features are bone pain, severe headache, dizziness and weakness, together with deafness, facial paralysis and blindness due to compression of the cochlear, facial and optic nerves, respectively.

Clinical features

The bones most frequently affected are the sacrum, spine, femora, skull, sternum and pelvis. Facial bone involvement occurs in the maxilla more frequently than the mandible. The affected maxillary alveolar ridge becomes widened and the palate flattened. Edentulous patients may complain of increasing tightness of their dentures due to the enlarging jaws, though the denture appears to contain and limit enlargement of the bone (Figure 8.3). The jaws expand to fill the space available, for example by filling in extraction spaces in the opposing jaw, but the expansion force is weaker than the normal muscle tone so that the jaw relationship is unaltered. Even in gross expansion the jaws are not forced apart, although the anterior alveolus may be visible and the lips stretched over the enlarged bone. The fact that the sinuses are not obliterated, even in advanced maxillary disease, must indicate that there is at least intermittent positive pressure within the sinus cavity (see Chapter 2).

The teeth may become hypercementosed and fused to sclerotic areas of bone. This makes extraction hazardous and large masses of bone may be unintentionally removed with the teeth. Forceps extraction may prove impossible and severe bleeding or osteomyelitis may follow.

Biochemical investigations are essential for diagnosis. The serum calcium and serum phosphate levels are usually within normal limits but the serum alkaline phosphatase is elevated to an extreme degree, particularly in the osteoblastic phase of the disease and when there is polyostotic involvement.

Radiographic features

The main features are decreased density in the early stages and sclerosis in the later stages. The loss of bony trabeculation and the irregular osteoblastic activity give the bone the characteristic 'cotton wool' appearance.

The disease is usually bilateral but may start unilaterally and resemble diffuse sclerosing osteomyelitis. The teeth show hypercementosis with loss of lamina dura. Root resorption is unusual, although it has been reported.

Treatment

Treatment with disodium etidronate or calcitonin is effective in arresting progress of the disease and alleviating symptoms.

Prognosis

Although the disease is chronic and progressive it is seldom the primary cause of death. The complications are due to the bony alterations and include pathological fractures, skeletal deformities and the visual and auditory problems due to encroachment on bony canals. The most common effect on the jaws is recalcitrant chronic infection, which occurs easily if the integrity of the thin, stretched overlying mucosa is breached by tooth extraction or minor trauma

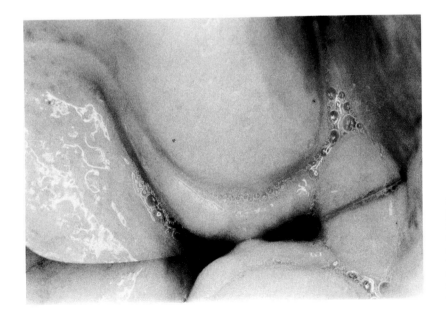

Figure 8.3 Maxillary tuberosity of a patient with Paget's disease of bone. A groove in the bone corresponding to the edge of the denture demarcates the ridge area, where the bone expansion has been contained by the denture, from the expanded tuberosity beyond its confines

(McGowan, 1974). The most serious recognized complication is osteosarcoma, which is 30 times more frequent in patients with Paget's disease over the age of 40 years than in unaffected individuals. The development of osteosarcoma may be related to the proliferative capacity of the diseased bone.

Cherubism

This is an uncommon disease affecting the jaws and, despite its previous synonyms (familial fibrous dysplasia of the jaws and hereditary fibrous dysplasia of the jaws), is not now regarded as fibrous dysplasia. The disease was first reported in 1933 by Jones, who coined the term 'cherubism' to describe the clinical and facial deformity of those affected.

Clinical features

Progressive painless symmetrical swelling of the jaws in early childhood produces the chubby face of a cherub. In severe cases involving the maxilla, the swellings cause the eyes to appear to be turned upwards, also contributing to the cherubic appearance. However, the maxilla is often unaffected and the vast majority of cases involve the mandible alone. The swelling begins at the age of 3 or 4 years and the deciduous teeth may be prematurely shed as early as 3 years of age. There is no pain or tenderness in the affected bones, although there may be enlargement of regional lymph nodes.

Growth is rapid for a few years then slows until puberty, sometimes regressing to produce a normal facial contour.

Radiological features

Extensive bilateral bone destruction is seen, with a multilocular appearance and perforation of the cortex. Teeth may be unerupted and displaced and some may appear to be floating in cyst-like spaces.

Treatment

As the disease shows natural regression in most cases, conservative management is indicated. Cosmetic surgical correction of the jaws can be carried out after puberty if necessary.

Benign tumours

Benign tumours in the sinus may arise from the lining as polyps and papillomas, from the bone as osteomas, or from the maxillary teeth as odontogenic tumours.

These lesions are notable for the lack of symptoms which they cause while contained within the sinus. They are often an incidental finding on radiographs taken for the diagnosis of sinusitis or dental disease. Some benign polyps or papillomas extend through the ostium into the nose causing obstruction there. Other lesions may come to light only after they have grown to such a size as to obliterate the sinus completely and expand beyond its confines.

Antral polyps

The thickened and folded mucosa in chronic sinusitis may form polyps, which are simply aggregations of oedematous submucous tissue covered in normal-appearing epithelium. They may arise from any part of the sinus wall and occasionally pass through the ostium to appear in the nose as an antrochoanal polyp. This form is found in young patients and is not associated with hypersensitivity or asthma like the majority of nasal polyps originating in the main from the ethmoid sinuses, and which exhibit a marked eosinophilia and high levels of immunoglobulins A and E. About 8% of patients with nasal polyps also suffer from asthma and, in addition, are hypersensitive to aspirin (Drake-Lee, 1987). Nasal polyps are removed by avulsion or snaring to relieve obstructive symptoms but, apart from the antrochoanal form, surgery for antral polyps *per se* is seldom justified. Antral polyps may prolapse through an oroantral fistula and are removed at closure (see Figure 5.7).

Antral papilloma

Squamous papillomas may occur in areas of squamous metaplasia in the nose and sinuses, as on any mucous surface, but a characteristic lesion which occurs only in this region is the so-called 'inverted' papilloma. The term describes the histological appearance, with deep invaginations of epithelium into the stroma, and there are also typically microscopic mucous cysts to be seen in the epithelium. They tend to recur after removal, though this is ascribed to technical difficulties in achieving total excision rather than exuberant growth potential. There is, however, considered to be a high potential for malignant change, estimated at 2–5% of cases (Cheeseman, 1987).

Hempenstall and Savage (1990) report a case of inverted papilloma which was discovered as a result of exploration of a non-healing discharging upper molar extraction socket.

Odontomes

Maxillary odontomes have been described in the sinuses (Shatz and Calderon, 1987). They are found incidentally by radiography or there may be symptoms from associated chronic infection (Figures 8.4 and 8.5). Removal is usually achieved by a Caldwell–Luc approach and is only difficult if the lesion is large.

Benign osteoblastoma

The benign osteoblastoma is an uncommon tumour which, as the name suggests, is characterized by the presence of numerous osteoblasts in a richly vascular stroma and the formation of bony, or at least osteoid tissue. The lesion may be considered as part of the spectrum of fibro-osseous conditions and must be distinguished from osteogenic sarcoma or giant cell lesions because it has a favourable prognosis. A helpful distinguishing feature is the surrounding thin shell of reactive cortical bone.

The maxillary sinus is a rare site for benign osteoblastoma, which is more commonly found in the spine or long bones, but a small number of cases has been

Figure 8.4 Infected odontome in the left maxillary sinus with a long associated history of chronic purulent discharge

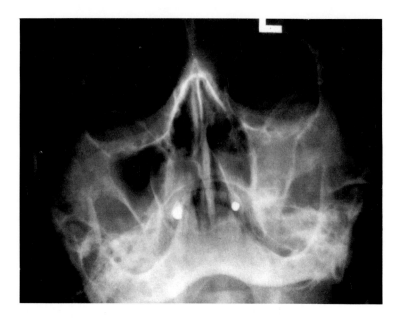

reported. The lesions have been discovered because of the symptoms produced by the expanding mass. Surgical excision is curative and because of the rich vascularity may be usefully preceded by arteriography and embolization to reduce blood flow into the lesion and consequent preoperative or postoperative haemorrhage (Osguthorpe and Hungerford, 1983).

The distinction between osteoblastomas and cementoblastomas is academic because their behaviour and clinical significance is identical. A case described as a giant cementoblastoma of the maxillary sinus was reported by Puterman *et al.* (1988).

Osteoma

The paranasal sinuses most frequently affected by this lesion are the frontal and ethmoid sinuses (Figure 8.6). Osteomas of the maxillary sinus do occur but they are very rare (Leopard, 1972).

The aetiology is unknown, although it is most likely that they are benign tumours of bone or hamartomas. Multiple osteomas of the facial bones are a feature of the Gardner syndrome and this possibility needs to be explored if more than one is detected radiologically. The diagnosis is well worth making so that attention can be given to the potentially malignant multiple polyps of the colon which, together with epidermoid cysts and desmoid tumours, are the other features of the syndrome.

Antroliths

While over 300 cases of rhinoliths found in the nasal passages have been published, the formation of calcified stones in the maxillary sinuses is far more unusual. Less than ten reports of antroliths have been published and most of these are single cases rather than series (Bowerman, 1969; Karges, Eversole and

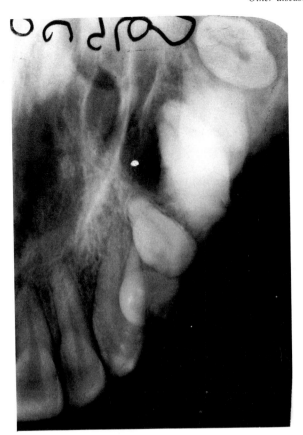

Figure 8.5 Odontome in the upper left first molar position which extended into the maxillary sinus. A large opening into the sinus which was created at removal was successfully closed by a buccal flap

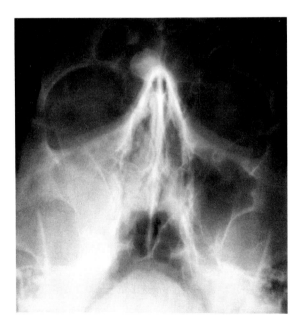

Figure 8.6 Osteoma of the right frontal sinus. An incidental finding on a radiograph taken to assist diagnosis of a right maxillary sinusitis and an unerupted third molar

Poindexter, 1971). Antroliths appear to form by a process of calcific accretion around a central nidus, which may be a small curd of natural secretion or a foreign body such as a dental dressing material, a seed or a fragment of paper, which has probably been inhaled. Rhinoliths form in the same way and are more frequent because of the greater accessibility of the nasal passages, particularly to the insertion of foreign bodies in childhood. It is likely that asymptomatic antroliths will be more frequently disclosed as the use of panoramic radiography increases (Jain and Frommer, 1982). The possibility of an antrolith must, however, be considered in the differential diagnosis of calcified masses within the antrum and in the identification and location of displaced dental root fragments. Antroliths have been removed because of diagnostic uncertainty but this should be resolvable by further radiography. Surgery is only really required if there are symptoms arising from associated chronic infection.

Ameloblastoma

Although much more common in the mandible (80%), ameloblastoma does occur in the maxilla and may rarely enlarge into the sinus, as in the cases described by Porter, Miller and Stratigos (1977) and by Keay *et al.* (1988).

Other rare tumours

Yusuf, Fajemisin and McWilliam (1989) removed a neurilemmoma from the maxillary sinus, Nam *et al.* (1988) a xanthoma in a patient with familial hypercholesterolaemia, and Salman *et al.* (1989) a granular cell tumour. A solitary plasmacytoma reported by Ilankovan, Moos and El-Attar (1990) was treated successfully by radiotherapy. Expansive lesions of the pterygopalatine fossa, such as a hydatid cyst, may displace the posterolateral wall of the sinus forwards (Akyildiz, Ozbilen and Goksu, 1991). This is also a characteristic diagnostic sign observed on lateral sinus radiographs of patients with juvenile angiofibroma (Lloyd and Phelps, 1986).

Tropical diseases

The antra may become involved in chronic nasal infections, which are most common in tropical countries and associated either with climatic conditions or malnourishment. Examples are rhinoschleroma in Egypt (Gamea, 1990), leprosy in the Indian subcontinent (Soni, 1989) and aspergillosis in Northern Sudan (De Foer, Fossion and Vaillant, 1990). Even myiasis (infestation with fly larvae) may extend to the sinuses (Duque, Marrugo and Valderrama, 1990).

Granulomatoses

Sarcoidosis, which is common in the nose in some populations, can affect the sinuses either primarily or in continuity with nasal lesions (Walker, Jones and Griffin, 1984). A single case of mycosis fungoides, a progressive reticular disorder first manifesting in skin, has been reported by Reynolds *et al.* (1981). The jaws and sinuses may be involved in the destruction caused by tertiary syphillis, gangosa or yaws (Weir, 1987) but neither tuberculosis nor actinomycosis appear to have been reported. Spiera, Lawson and Weinrauch (1988) report a patient with Wegener's granulomatosis affecting the sinuses; the granulomatosis was completely eliminated by treatment with co-trimoxazole.

References

Akyildiz, A. N., Ozbilen, M. S. and Goksu, N. (1991) Hydatid cyst of the pterygopalatine fossa. *Journal of Oral and Maxillofacial Surgery*, **49**, 87–88

Bowerman, J. E. (1969) The maxillary antrolity. *Journal of Laryngology*, **83**, 873–882

Cheeseman, A. D. (1987) Non-healing granulomata and lesions of the nose and sinus. In *Scott-Brown's Otolaryngology*, Vol. 4, 5th edn (eds I. S. Mackay and T. R. Bull), Butterworth–Heinemann, Oxford, chap. 18

Darlow, L. D., Murphy, J. B., Berrios, R. J., Park, Y. and Feldman, R. S. (1988) Arteriovenous malformation of the maxillary sinus: an unusual clinical presentation. *Oral Surgery, Oral Medicine, Oral Pathology*, **66**, 21–23

De Foer, C., Fossion, E. and Vaillant, J. M. (1990) Sinus aspergillosis. *Journal of Cranio-Maxillo-Facial Surgery*, **18**, 33–40

Drake-Lee, A. B. (1987) Nasal polyps. In *Scott-Brown's Otolaryngology*, Vol. 4, 5th edn (eds I. S. Mackay and T. R. Bull), Butterworth–Heinemann, Oxford, chap. 9

Duque, C. S., Marrugo, G. and Valderrama, R. (1990) Otolaryngic manifestations of myiasis. *Ear, Nose and Throat Journal*, **69**, 619–622

Gamea, A. M. (1990) Role of endoscopy in diagnosing scleroma in its uncommon sites. *Journal of Laryngology and Otology*, **104**, 619–621

Harris, M. (1993) Central giant cell granulomas of the jaws regress with calcitonin therapy. *British Journal of Oral and Maxillofacial Surgery*, **31**, 89–94

Hempenstall, P. D. and Savage, N. W. (1990) Inverted papilloma of the maxillary sinus: an unusual cause of a non-healing extraction socket. Case report. *Australian Dental Journal*, **35**, 241–244

Ilankovan, V., Moos, K. F. and El-Attar, A. (1990) Intramedullary plasma cell tumours. *International Journal of Oral and Maxillofacial Surgery*, **19**, 323–326

Jain, R. K. and Frommer, H. H. (1982) Incidental finding of antroliths in panoramic radiography. *New York State Dental Journal*, **48**, 530–531

Karges, M. A., Eversole, L. R. and Poindexter, B. J. Jr (1971) Antrolith: report of a case and review of the literature. *Journal of Oral Surgery*, **29**, 812–814

Keay, D. G., Small, M., Kerr, A. I. G. and McLaren, K. (1988) Ameloblastoma presenting as nasal obstruction. *Journal of Laryngology and Otology*, **102**, 530–533

Leopard, P. J. (1972) Osteoma of the maxillary sinus. *British Journal of Oral Surgery*, **10**, 73–77

Lloyd, G. A. S. and Phelps, P. D. (1986) Juvenile angiofibroma: imaging by magnetic resonance, CT and conventional techniques. *Clinical Otolaryngology*, **11**, 247–259

McGowan, D. A. (1974) Clinical problems in Paget's disease affecting the jaws. *British Journal of Oral Surgery*, **11**, 230–235

Maran, A. G. D. and Kerr, A. I. G. (1990) What's new in surgery: otolaryngology. *Journal of the Royal College of Surgeons of Edinburgh*, **35**, 140–143

Mossey, P. and Sandham, J. (1989) Maxillonasal dysplasia, mandibular retrognathia and cleft palate *Angle Orthodontist*, **59**, 257–262

Nam, M. H., Grande, J. P., Chin-yang, L., Kottke, B. A., Pineda, A. A. and Weiland, L. M. (1988) Familial hypercholesterolemia with unusual foamy histocytes. Report of a case with myelopthisic anaemia and xanthoma of the maxillary sinus. *American Journal of Clinical Pathology*, **89**, 556–561

Osguthorpe, J. D. and Hungerford, G. D. (1983) Benign osteoblastoma of the maxillary sinus. *Head and Neck Surgery*, **6**, 605–609

Porter, J., Miller, R. and Stratigos, G. T. (1977) Ameloblastoma of the maxilla. *Oral Surgery, Oral Medicine, Oral Pathology*, **44**, 34–38

Puterman, M., Fliss, M., Sidi, J. and Zirkin, H. (1988) Giant cementoblastoma simulating a peridental infection. *Journal of Laryngology and Otology*, **102**, 264–266

Reynolds, W. R., Feldman, M. I., Bricout, P. B. and Potdar, G. G. (1981) Mycosis fungoides in the maxillary sinus and oral cavity: report of two cases. *Journal of Oral Surgery*, **39**, 373–377

Salman, R. A., Leonetti, J. A., Salman, L. and Chaudhry, A. P. (1989) Adult benign granular cell tumour of the maxilla. *Journal of Oral Pathology and Medicine*, **18**, 517–519

Schwartz, D. T. and Alpert, M. (1964) The malignant transformation of fibrous dysplasia. *American Journal of the Medical Sciences*, **247**, 35–54

Shafer, W. G., Hine, M. K. and Levy, B. M. (1983) *A Textbook of Oral Pathology*, 4th edn, W. B. Saunders, Philadelphia

Shatz, A. and Calderon, S. (1987) Complex odontoma in the maxillary sinus. An unusual presentation. *Annals of Dentistry*, **46**, 38–40

Sheppard, L. M. and Mickelson, S. A. (1990) Haemangiomas of the nasal septum and paranasal sinuses. *Henry Ford Hospital Medical Journal*, **38**, 25–27

Smith, P. G., Marrogi, A. J. and Delfino, J. J. (1990) Multifocal central giant cell lesions of the maxillofacial skeleton: a case report. *Journal of Oral and Maxillofacial Surgery*, **48**, 300–305

Soni, N. K. (1989) Antroscopic study of the maxillary antrum in lepromatous leprosy. *Journal of Laryngology and Otology*, **103**, 502–503

Spiera, H., Lawson, W. and Weinrauch, H. (1988) Wegener's granulomatosis treated with sulphamethoxazole–trimethoprim. Report of a case. *Archives of Internal Medicine*, **148**, 2065–2066

Tanner, H. C., Dahlin, D. C. and Childs, D. S. (1961) Sarcoma complicating fibrous dysplasia. Probable role of radiation therapy. *Oral Surgery, Oral Medicine, Oral Pathology*, **14**, 837–846

Walker, A. N., Jones, P. F. and Griffin, W. L. (1984) Residents page: Pathologic Quiz Case 1. Sinonasal Sarcoidosis. *Archives of Otolaryngology*, **110**, 132–134

Watson, L. and Faccini, J. M. (1976) Metabolic diseases of the jaws. In: *Scientific Foundations of Dentistry*, edited by B. Cohen and I. R. H. Kramer. William Heinemann Medical Books, pp. 573–581

Weir, N. (1987) Acute and chronic inflammations of the nose. In *Scott-Brown's Otolaryngology*, Vol. 4, 5th edn (eds I. S. Mackay and T. R. Bull), Butterworth–Heinemann, Oxford, chap. 8

Yusuf, H., Fajemisin, O. A. and McWilliam, L. J. (1989) Neurilemmoma involving the maxillary sinus: a case report. *British Journal of Oral and Maxillofacial Surgery*, **27**, 506–511

Chapter 9

Ethical and medicolegal considerations

While the dentist clearly has a professional duty to recognize, diagnose and give advice on treatment for anomalies, diseases or disorders of the teeth, jaws and mouth, how far does this interest properly extend? How much treatment should be undertaken of conditions not traditionally regarded as the province of the dental surgeon, whether generalist or specialist, and indeed how much of a duty is there to act in general health screening? The subject of this book is an anatomical interface area, and these questions are particularly pertinent to the problems which have been dealt with in the previous chapters. The principles of the Hippocratic oath have guided physicians and surgeons for centuries and remain central to medical ethics. One of these principles is that the treatment should do the patient no harm, and this, coupled with the principle of 'do as you would be done by' (sometimes less selfishly expressed as 'how would you treat this patient if he or she were your parent, partner or child?'), provides the conscientious practitioner with all the guidance needed for ethical behaviour. Such ethical behaviour in itself is the best possible defence to criticism, be it in conversation or in court. Misfortune cannot be avoided, and occasional lapses of skill, care or understanding are inevitable. The practitioner's duty is to strive to avoid them, but, provided the response is honest and caring, there need be no feelings of guilt, nor will there necessarily be culpability in case of failure. In an area of myriad complexities, such as human therapy, only the arrogant and ignorant can be unaware of the limitations of their own knowledge and that of others.

A dentist who recognizes the presence of disease in the maxillary sinus must be sufficiently knowledgeable to assess its significance in general terms. Where this is trivial, for example a finding on a radiograph of a small mucous cyst of the sinus, then deciding on the action to be taken is relatively easy. The patient can be told that there is a curious but harmless abnormality present, and that may be the end of the matter. However, even in these circumstances some patients become alarmed and the clinician may regret mentioning the matter. It is better to be guided by prediction of the patient's likely reaction than by fear of legal action, if the practitioner chooses not to divulge the information. At the other extreme, in the case of a tentative diagnosis of a malignant tumour in the sinus, it is imperative that the patient be told, but the difficulty is in deciding what is to be said. It is proper to describe such a lesion as, for example, a 'blocked' sinus requiring treatment, to advise that a specialist colleague should be consulted without delay, and to make arrangements for such a consultation. It is wise to check that the appointment is kept, to become firm in persuasion if the patient is reluctant, and perhaps to enlist the support of the medical general practitioner by informing him or her of the suspicion. Some patients may realize that cancer is a possibility, or may even be convinced of their imminent death. Discussion should then be more frank and should stress a hopeful prognosis, provided effective treatment is accepted without delay. Fortunately, this fear is very unlikely to occur spontaneously in malignant maxillary sinus disease, but recently the authors had to deal with the mother of a dental ancillary worker who had undergone a radical mastectomy and was receiving chemotherapy for the treatment of secondary disease. She presented to us, after a long delay, with marked swelling of the left cheek which she correctly assumed to be related to spread of tumour to her maxilla. She was well aware of her disease and its prognosis but delayed seeking advice about the facial swelling because she feared having surgery which would leave her disfigured. She was delighted to be reassured that this need not be so and indeed had some palliative radiotherapy to the area which held the tumour in check during her terminal illness.

On less weighty matters, there seems little harm in a dentist undertaking simple treatment such as prescribing analgesics, antibiotics and nasal decongestant drops for a patient in whom he has diagnosed an acute sinusitis. It is best, however, to advise the patient to seek follow-up advice from a physician, as the episode is unlikely to be the last. In any case, the current regulations governing the remuneration of dentists in UK health service general practice do not recognize such activity!

The dentist, however, does have a clear moral and ethical duty to deal promptly and efficiently with relatively common complications of dental treatment. Oroantral communication following tooth extraction is a clear-cut example, particularly so since there is ample evidence that delay is detrimental in such cases. That is not to say that every dentist must close every communication immediately, however desirable this might be. If realistic appraisal of skill, experience and circumstances suggests that the patient would be better served by urgent reference to a colleague, then that is what should be arranged.

Consideration of this problem also raises the difficult judgement of the duty of the dentist to warn the patient before extraction of the possibility of antral perforation. It would be unreasonable to warn every patient of every possible complication of the surgery to which they are about to submit themselves: this would be both tedious and alarming. On the other hand, such a warning is prudent when a complication is more likely than usual to occur and when there is reason, on the basis of the history or the radiographs, to anticipate it.

Complications of dental practice involving the maxillary sinus are not currently a frequent or substantial medicolegal problem in the UK, and recent enquiry from the professional malpractice defence societies failed to turn up any cases.

The maxillary sinus is a relatively large anatomical area which lies near to the upper dentition. Its involvement in dental treatment may be an unfortunate nuisance, but it need not be a surgical disaster. To get in is easy – to get out successfully requires knowledge and skill!

Appendices

Appendix 1 (see Figure 1.9)
Opened pyramid showing some
internal and external relations of the
maxillary sinus. Instructions for
making up a three-dimensional
model can be found on p.159

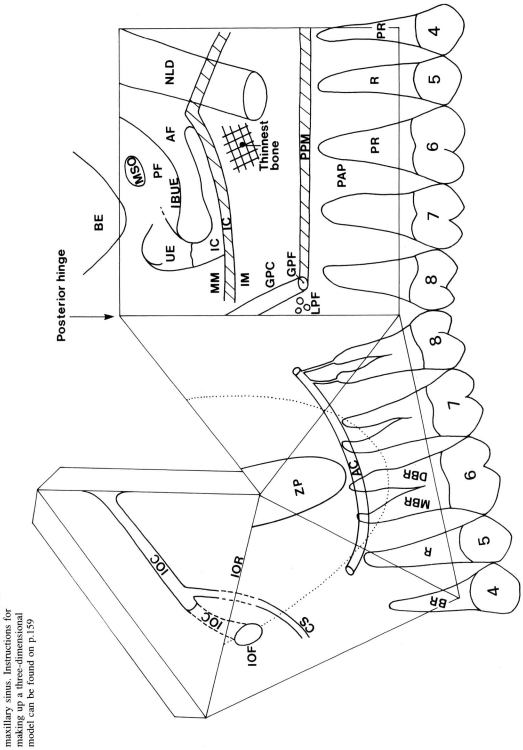

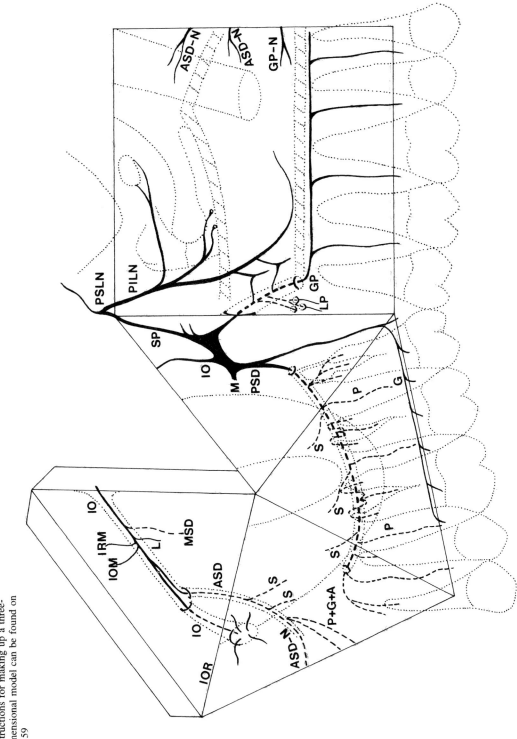

Appendix 2 (see Figure 1.17)
Opened pyramid showing arteries
related to the maxillary sinus.
Instructions for making up a three-
dimensional model can be found on
p.159

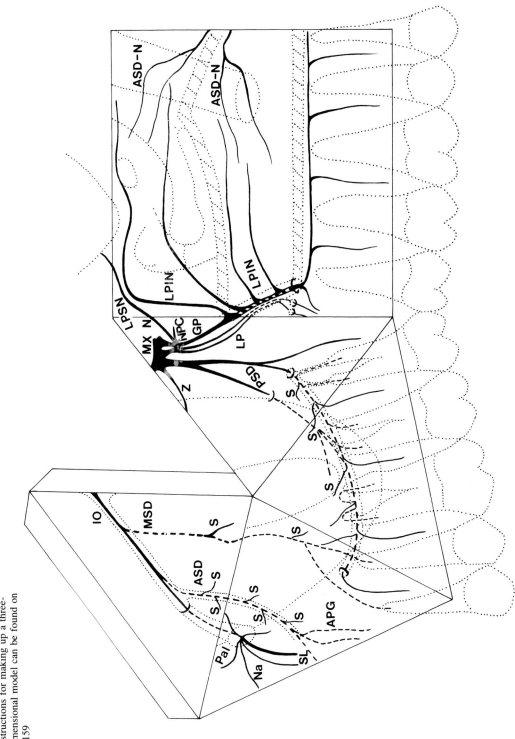

Appendix 3 (see Figure 1.18)
Opened pyramid showing nerves
associated with the maxillary sinus.
Instructions for making up a three-
dimensional model can be found on
p.159

Instructions for making up a three-dimensional model

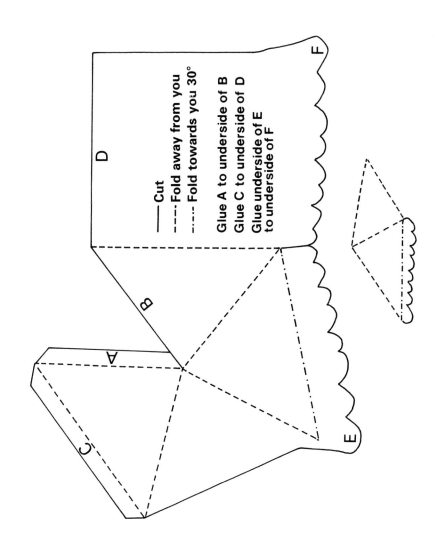

Glue A to underside of B
Glue C to underside of D
Glue underside of E
to underside of F

———— Cut
- - - - Fold away from you
- · - · - Fold towards you 30°

D

B

A

C

E

F

Index